THE MIGRAINE REVOLUTION

Examines the importance of food and chemical allergy in migraine, and points the way to a healthier lifestyle which will lessen the chance of continued migraine attacks.

D0956623

THE
MIGRAINE
REVOLUTION

The
New Drug-Free
Solution

Dr John Mansfield

THORSONS PUBLISHING GROUP
Wellingborough * New York

First published August 1986
Second Impression August 1986

© DR J. R. MANSFIELD 1986

*All rights reserved. No part of this book may be reproduced or utilized
in any form or by any means, electronic or mechanical, including
photocopying, recording or by any information storage and retrieval
system, without permission in writing from the Publisher.*

British Library Cataloguing in Publication Data

Mansfield, J. R.
    The migraine revolution: the new drug-free
    solution
    1. Migraine — Nutritional aspects
    I. Title
    616.8'57071   RC392

    ISBN 0-7225-1314-3

Printed and bound in Great Britain

CONTENTS

	Page
Foreword by Dr R. Finn	7
Introduction: Migraine is Curable	9
A Case History: Jenny's Migraines	13
Chapter	
1. Migraine — the Problem	19
2. Food Allergy and Its Historical Development	22
3. Chemical Allergy and Its Historical Development	37
4. The Elimination Diet	44
5. The Management of Food and Chemical Allergy	54
6. The Role of Alcohol, Smoking, the Pill and Ergotamine in Migraine	62
7. The Intestinal Thrush Factor	71
8. Neutralization and Desensitization to Foods	86
9. Desensitization and Other Techniques for Dealing with Inhaled Allergies	94
10. Evidence that Neutralization Works	101
11. Other Methods of Diagnosing and Treating Food Allergies	109
12. The Migraine Trials	118
13. The Roots of Allergy	129
14. Accepting These Concepts	143
15. Summary and Conclusion	148
Useful Addresses	151
Further Reading	155
Index	157

DEDICATION

To my nurses and technicians at the Burgh Wood Clinic who have given me enormous help and support over the past few years.

FOREWORD

Migraine is often associated with visual symptoms such as flashing lights. Micropsia is an extremely rare visual manifestation of migraine in which all objects appear to be very small. An Oxford mathematician called Charles Dodgson suffered from this very unusual symptom and from his experiences, he conceived of the 'little people' whom he used as the basis for *Alice's Adventures in Wonderland*, which he wrote under the pseudonym of Lewis Carroll.

Such a fortunate outcome is unusual in migraine, which causes much human misery. It is responsible for more loss of time from work than industrial disputes and thus, costs the country large amounts of money. Although a disease which causes much suffering, it is not usually a serious condition. Nevertheless, suicide has been reported in some very severe cases and the taking of large quantities of pain-killing drugs over many years can occasionally lead to kidney damage with serious consequences. Conventional drug treatment is of only limited value and it is reasonable that severe sufferers should explore alternative approaches. There is now good evidence that modification of diet can help many patients with migraine. Simple modifications of diet can be carried out by the patient on his own, but as the author points out, more complicated exclusion diets and other measures described in this book, should only be carried out under expert medical supervision; and it is also essential that other causes of headache should be excluded by a medical practitioner.

Dr John Mansfield is one of the pioneers of allergy research in this country and his book is to be warmly recommended to all those who wish to learn more about this new approach to migraine.

RONALD FINN M.D., F.R.C.P.
Consultant Physician
Royal Liverpool Hospital
Liverpool L7 8XP

INTRODUCTION
MIGRAINE IS CURABLE

For several years a large number of doctors in Great Britain, the USA and Australia have been convinced that they knew what was causing migraine and how to cure a very high proportion of patients suffering from this disease. Their claims were met with reactions ranging from scepticism to ridicule by most of their medical colleagues. However, in 1983 and 1984 there were several papers published in eminent medical journals, all of which have almost totally substantiated these claims.

Some of this work has clearly demonstrated that food allergy is the main single cause of migraine and that it accounts for between 80-90 per cent of this problem. The other work has demonstrated that there is an effective method for desensitizing patients to food allergies. As many of the foods involved with migraine are very difficult to avoid, desensitization is usually a vitally necessary part of the treatment. With the demonstration that most migraine is due to food allergy and with the further proof that food desensitization is effective, I have given the book the rather provocative title that it has. Although the title is provocative, it is now scientifically demonstrable.

On 15 October 1983, *The Lancet* published a paper entitled, 'Is Migraine Food Allergy? A double-blind controlled trial of oligo-antigenic diet treatment (low-risk allergy diet).' The authors were Professor Soothill and his colleagues at the Department of Neurology and Immunology at the Hospital for Sick Children (Great Ormond Street) and the Institue of Child Health. They summarize their trial by stating that 93 per cent of 88 children with severe frequent migraine recovered on a low-risk allergy diet. Foods causing migraine were then identified by slowly reintroducing the foods back into the children's diet and noting the adverse reactions. To counteract the possibility that the children may have been psychologically reacting to these foods, the reactions in forty of the patients were then checked by double-blind controlled tests. These tests consisted of again giving the children foods which had already been implicated in causing their migraine, but disguised amongst other foods. Tins of food mixtures were made up, some of which had foods thought to be allergenic to the child, others containing foods thought not to be allergenic to the child. Neither the child nor the nurse who was administering the food knew which mixtures contained the known offending foods. When the code was broken at the end of the trial, it was discovered that the children reacted to the mixtures containing the items to which they were thought to be allergic, but not to the others. This trial was not the first trial to demonstrate the relationship of food allergy and migraine, but because so many double-blind controlled studies were done and because it came from such an eminent research institution, it finally proved this theory beyond all reasonable doubt. There are few concepts in medicine which relate to cause and effect which are now as well established as this. I will go later into more detail about this particular trial and ones that preceded and followed it, as there are lots of implications which should be brought out. Later in this book it will be demonstrated that although migraine is predominantly a food-allergy problem, in some patients the picture is complicated by chemicals in foods, inhalant allergies, nutritional problems and intestinal thrush.

Knowing that someone's migraines are caused by specific food allergies sometimes does not help them in itself if these foods are major items in the diet, which can be exceedingly difficult to avoid. Hence, I and a number of allergists now make widespread use of food desensitization which enables the patient to eat the food to which he is allergic without adverse response. In Chapter 8 a series of double-blind studies are described, which substantiate that this is an effective and reliable technique. Also in this chapter there is a brief outline of the technique itself, its uses and its limitations.

As this book is aimed at both physicians and laymen, there is also a description of an elimination dietary procedure which can be carried out. Elimination dieting is not easy and patients need a considerable degree of instruction as to how this procedure can be accomplished. Some people with mild to moderate migraine may utilize the information in this book to sort out their own migraine problems. If they do so, I should emphasize that they should check with their own GPs first that they are suffering from simple migraine or headaches and not some organic lesion. In my experience, most people need support and advice while going through these procedures and need someone to sort out the problems as they arise. As these problems tend to be multiple and severe in patients with severe and frequent migraine, I would not advise people with such problems to attempt this on their own. Various allergy organizations, such as Action Against Allergy, Chemical Victims, etc., whose addresses are at the back of this book, usually know of physicians who are experienced in these techniques. Futhermore, many people require desensitization, and if they do, medical help will obviously be necessary. In the chapter on the roots of allergy, there are some answers to the questions of why people acquire these food and chemical allergies and why they occur at particular times of life.

Finally, I outline what prospects there are of these ideas being incorporated into everyday medical practice and what hurdles have to be overcome first.

This book is written on one hand for lay people and on the other hand for a whole range of health-care professionals. There is the inherent danger in this of falling between two stools. I hope the lay readers will excuse me when I become a little technical at times and that the medically-qualified readers will do the same when the account is couched in more lay terminology.

A CASE HISTORY
JENNY'S MIGRAINES

Jenny Thompson was 29 when she first came to see me, an attractive, intelligent lady accompanied by her husband Jim, a successful young accountant. She told me that she was about 16 when she first noticed some headaches, but by the time she was 20 her migraines had started in earnest. At that time they were occurring about one per month. She tried taking the contraceptive pill when she was 20, which caused the migraines to become more frequent and severe. After a few months and having unsuccessfully tried three different brands, she reluctantly gave up this method of contraception. By the time she was 22, her headaches were now fairly regularly coming at two per month, one of which nearly always occurred in the day or two prior to her period. When Jenny was 25 she married Jim, who had been her regular boy-friend for the preceding three years. Her parents hoped that her marriage would help her headaches and migraine and her occasional mild bouts of depression but this hope was not to be realized, as the migraines, if anything, became a bit worse and she became more troubled with general fatigue and occasional depression.

Her first child, a son, was born when she was 27 and after the birth she became unexpectedly depressed. The hospital and her GP both diagnosed post-natal depresion and she was given a month's course of antidepressant tablets which gradually appeared to relieve the condition. She, however, remained much more fatigued than ever before in her life, a situation which she initially put down to the stress of feeding the baby during the night. The migraines were now even more frequent and often occurred at weekly intervals. Tranquillizers, antidepressants and migraine-preventive tablets were all tried with only marginal benefit. By now the slim figure of which she had been so proud was a thing of the past and, despite frequent crash diets, she had difficulty in keeping her weight down to 10 stone, while as a teenager she had never been above 9 stone.

Another 18 months later she had her second baby, also a boy, followed by an even worse post-natal depression, quite severe fatigue and severe migraines. She had an ongoing malaise and spent about one day per week in bed, suffering from the severe migraines. Dinner parties were inevitably followed by a migraine, as was any drink of spirits, although she seemed to be able to tolerate wine. Long journeys almost always provoked migraine, especially if a lot of traffic was encountered on the way. Her interest in sexual relationships with her husband, whom she still loved, had deteriorated alarmingly and was now worrying both of them.

As her health was becoming such a problem, she and Jim together went to see her GP to review the whole situation. He was an excellent young and enthusiastic doctor, the junior partner in the local group practice. After reviewing her whole case history, he admitted that all the drug treatment that she had tried had been only of marginal benefit and that her bathroom was now beginning to resemble a chemist's shop. He told them that he had just been reading details of several clinical trials that had been conducted at London teaching hospitals, which had demonstrated that most migraines appeared to be related to commonly eaten foods. Jenny told him that she had tried omitting cheese, chocolate, citrus fruits and red wine, but that this had made no difference to her problem. She had, however, noticed that chocolate did seem to be one cause of her migraines, but omitting it did not seem to ease the problem. Her GP explained that the trials had shown that commonly eaten foods like wheat, milk, eggs, yeast and sugar seemed to be the most frequent foods implicated. He explained that the foods involved varied enormously from one patient to another and needed to be sorted out either by an elimination diet or by some other technique for detecting food allergies. He gave her a referral to my clinic, where she consulted me a few weeks later.

During this consultation I told her I was particularly interested in her history of chronic fatigue, which is a major feature of food allergy. I found her story of severe responses to certain alcoholic beverages encouraging, as we know that reactions to such specific alcoholic beverages represent 'food allergy in a jet-propelled vehicle' — see Chapter 6. I also found, after some direct questioning, that she had a history of car sickness as a child, although she had had no problem with sickness in ships, planes and trains. The car sickness faded out in her early teens, but was replaced by headaches on car journeys. I explained that both the nausea and later the headaches were probably due to sensitivity to petrol fumes and the body's response to this sensitivity had changed with the passing years. I felt that most of Jenny's symptoms were, however, due to food allergy, which could best be sorted out by an elimination diet. She asked me if the food allergy could be identified by skin test or by blood test. I replied that ordinary prick tests for food allergy were useless and that intradermal provocative skin testing for food allergies using it as a diagnostic tool had some drawbacks. However, I told her that I did use it, for example, when time was at a premium but that it could work out rather expensive. The various types of blood test I consider inaccurate.

I suggested that Jenny should restrict her diet to lamb, cod, trout, salmon, pears, carrots, parsnips, turnips, swedes and courgettes for 5½ days with only bottled spring water to drink. I told her she could use sunflower oil for frying or basting and sea salt for flavouring. She was warned that when she started this diet she would, if she had one of the usual 'masked' allergies, have a withdrawal reaction leading usually to a major migraine, starting on the first day of the diet and lasting for up to three or four days.

When she returned to see me on the sixth day of her diet, she related somewhat ruefully that she had indeed had a horrible migraine starting at lunch-time on the first day of the diet, which was particularly severe on the evening of the first day and on the second day, followed by lessening intensity on days three and four. Her fatigue was awful on the second and third day and, in fact, she had spent most of the second day in bed. After the fourth day there was a marked improvement in this fatigue. To her surprise, she found that her muscles, especially those of her thighs, buttocks and lower back, ached as if she had had the 'flu. This eased off late on the fifth day.

When Jenny saw me on the sixth day her eyes were sparkling and she could hardly contain her enthusiasm for the changes that had occurred in the preceding 48 hours. She told me that she felt enormously better and that her constant fatigue had now disappeared. Her mind felt clearer than it had done for years. To her total delight she had also lost 7 lb weight in 5½ days and the puffiness which had marred her face had now disappeared.

I told her that she had had a classic withdrawal reaction and I was now certain that food allergy was her main problem. Now all we had to do was to reintroduce foods selectively back into her diet one at a time to identify which foods caused her to react. In the next seven days we introduced about twenty foods, all with a low risk of producing allergy. She passed all these foods with flying colours and by now her diet was quiet wide and substantial.

Later, when Jenny tried wheat, her extreme well-being rapidly deteriorated. Wheat is, like all the cereals, a food which we spend two days on testing, as it is very slowly absorbed and characteristically shows a rather sluggish reaction. By the first evening she began to notice that her old fatigue was coming back and the next morning she woke up with a mild headache. By lunch-time on the second day she had a full-blown migraine which continued for the next 1½ days, although she had stopped eating wheat by lunch-time on the second day. She had similar reactions with corn, oats, rye and malt, indicating a general cereal sensitivity. I told her that it was now obvious as to why she reacted to alcoholic beverages because both of her favourite tipples, Scotch and gin, are made from cereals (Scotch always and gin sometimes).

Except while reacting to these foods Jenny had continued to remain well, but of course the continued avoidance of such foods is very difficult and expensive. Accordingly, I offered her densensitization to her cereals. It was explained that one afternoon of skin testing would be required to determine the neutralizing levels for her food problems. To determine the suspected petrol/diesel inhalant problems would probably take another hour or so on the following day. Once her neutralizing levels to these foods and inhalants had been determined, these specific levels would be made up into desensitizing solutions which could either be taken by sublingual drops (particularly for the inhalants) or minute subcutaneous injections (preferably for the food). The injections would be taken on alternate days and administered by a small microneedle which the patient could use herself. Usually as soon as this treatment is initiated, the patient is able to consume the foods to which he or she is allergic without any adverse effect. After two or three years of such treatment the patient will be desensitized and then be able to eat the foods to which he or she is sensitive without problem.

In the three years since her 'sort out' Jenny has continued to remain perfectly well. She has only had two minor migraines after car journeys, when she forgot to take her petrol neutralizing drops. Nowadays the depression and fatigue are only a distant unpleasant memory.

This case history has been selected not because it is extraordinary, but because it is a classic run-of-the-mill case, typical of many we see every week at our clinic. There are countless Jenny Thompsons in modern-day society and most of them can now be helped by methods such as those described in this book.

1.
MIGRAINE — THE PROBLEM

It has been claimed by many authorities that migraine causes more suffering in toto than any other human affliction. It has been known and written about since early civilization. In fact, it is one of the oldest diseases known to man.

The incidence is world-wide and the only people who appear unaffected are peoples such as the bushmen of Africa. However, even these peoples, when they move into townships and start eating Westernized food, rapidly lose their immunity. In Great Britain, it is estimated that over five million people suffer from migraine at some time in their lives. The incidence is considerably higher in women and there are estimates that approximately 20 per cent of the adult female population suffer from migraine at some time or another. Millions of working days are lost every year because of this complaint and its economic cost to the country is quite enormous.

Famous people in the past who have suffered badly from this complaint include Lewis Carroll, Rudyard Kipling, Sigmund Freud, George Eliot and Joan of Arc. The most famous sufferer in the present day is Princess Margaret, and the British Migraine Trust Clinic in Charterhouse Square is named after her.

What is Migraine?
Classically, a migraine is described as a headache accompanied by nausea and often vomiting. In some sufferers these complaints are preceded by what are termed fortification spectra. These are visual symptoms and the patient perceives either zig-zag lines or bright flashing lights. Sometimes these symptoms can be really severe and parts of the field of vision become completely blotted out. Some people feel as if they

are going blind. Usually, when the fortification spectra disappear, they give way to headache, nausea and vomiting. Although this book is written predominantly about migraine, I must emphasize that it has been one of the mistakes in the past to consider this condition in isolation. Most migraine sufferers also at times suffer from non-migrainous headaches and these headaches are often minor versions of the more severe migraine. There is a whole spectrum of headaches from minor to moderate to severe to full-blown migraine, and it is probable that the cause of each of these items is similar. Similarly, most patients also suffer from other conditions, such as fatigue, depression, episodes of fast-beating heart, swelling of the ankles, abnormal blood-pressure and overweight. Commonly, a migraine sufferer will experience one or other of these symptoms as well as his/her migraine, and these conditions are all tied up with the basic allergy problem. Migraine is, therefore, just one expression of man's inability to adapt successfully to his environment, using the term in its widest sense to include foods, chemicals and inhalants.

Another variety of migraine is termed abdominal migraine. This is a condition in which the patient suffers from recurrent abdominal pain, usually with nausea and vomiting, which on investigation is found to have no demonstrable organic cause. This is thus thought of as a 'headache of the stomach'.

A comparatively rare variant of migraine is cluster migraine, a condition in which the patient is free of symptoms for many months entirely, but then suddenly develops migraine symptoms day after day, often for several weeks on end.

Current Treatment
The current treatment of migraine is predominantly symptomatic, for though certain food items, such as cheese, chocolate, citrus fruits and red wine, have for many years been recognized as being able to precipitate migraine, the total elimination of these items from a migraineur's diet will only stop migraine completely in about 2 per cent of cases. The reason for this (which in short is that these foods are not the common food allergens) will become apparent later.

The current drug treatment for migraine divides into the drugs which are purely suppressive, and three that are possibly preventive. There is currently a huge range of pain-killers on the market, of which the most well-known are aspirin, codeine, solpadeine and paracetamol. These drugs, of course, do nothing other than relieve pain. A more specific anti-migraine drug is ergotamine tartrate, which is present in such medications as Cafergot and Migril, and in some patients this can have a fairly marked effect on aborting an attack if taken early enough. However, some patients with frequent migraine can become heavily dependent on this drug, which has well-known toxic effects if taken in excess and there is evidence, which will be discussed later, that frequent dosing with ergotamine tartrate can eventually lead to the ergotamine itself being part of the cause of the migraine.

Tranquillizers and two drugs, Dixarit (clonidine hydrochloride) and Deseril (Methylsergide), are all claimed to have some effect on reducing the frequency and severity of migraine attacks. The effect of tranquillizers in my experience is fairly minimal, but Dixarit reduces the sensitivity of the blood vessels to adverse stimuli. It was originally introduced in 1969 and is claimed to reduce the severity and frequency of attacks in up to 30 per cent of cases. Deseril is a fairly potent drug and can help to some degree in the very severe cases for which it is normally reserved. It has several rather nasty possible side-effects and is rarely used because of this.

All the above medications are very limited in their value and none of them really stop the condition. Futhermore, none tell us anything about what causes migraine. Most sufferers end up by taking simple pain-killers and putting as brave a face as they can on their condition. The new approaches described in this book can radically alter this outlook.

2

FOOD ALLERGY AND
ITS HISTORICAL DEVELOPMENT

The idea that foods can produce abnormal reactions has an extremely long history and has always been the subject of considerable medical interest. The aphorism that 'one man's meat is another man's poison' has been attributed to Lucretius, who lived about one hundred years BC. For many centuries dietary manipulations were one of the main areas of medical endeavour, but as interest in pharmacology grew in the past century, this concept was relegated to the backwaters of medicine. It is now being demonstrated that this was a considerable oversight. In this century, the first person to draw attention to the influence that food has in disease processes was Dr Francis Hare, an Australian psychiatrist who ran a clinic for alcoholics in Beckenham, Kent. In 1905 he published a huge two-volume work called *The Food Factor in Disease.* His work showed an amazing amount of knowledge and insight into the subject and he cited many individual case histories of patients who had responded to these ideas. Some of the patients he described had suffered from head pain or migraine.

Allergy Defined
The concept that an illness was an interraction between external environmental factors and individual capacity to resist them begain to emerge at about this time. Immunology took into account this individual response to external excitants and in 1906 an Austrian physician, Clement von Pirquet, coined the term 'allergy'. The term was derived from two Greek words and meant altered reactivity. In other words, an allergy was a response to a substance which affected one individual but not another.

The use or supposed misuse of the term allergy has caused

the most amazing schisms amongst various physicians working with patients who have adverse reactions to foods. Most immunologists assert that when von Pirquet coined the term allergy he meant it to cover only those reactions in which a specific immunologic (antigen-antibody) reaction could be demonstrated. A colleague of von Pirquet, Dr Doerr, in a paper published three years later, quite definitely widened the use of the term allergy to cover every form of altered reactivity, whether an underlying antigen-antibody reaction could be shown or not.

However, further study of von Pirquet's writing showed that he realized that a condition that should produce immunity can sometimes produce supersensitivity, and that immunity and supersensitivity can be 'most closely related'. He concluded that it was difficult or impossible to dissociate these terms and that there was a need for a generalized term which prejudiced nothing. He later stated that, 'for the general concept of a changed reactivity, I propose the term 'allergy''. Comparing the terms 'allergen' with 'antigen', he asserted that the term 'allergen' was more far-reaching and could include substances that lead to supersensitivity but not to production of antibodies. He thus meant the word 'allergy' to be a term which would prejudice nothing and could cover reactions which had no known immunologic basis. Because of this I unashamedly use the word 'allergy' freely throughout this text.

The next major contribution to the field came from Albert Rowe, a physician in California. He devised a series of elimination diets which left out whole groups of foods one at a time. He later fed such groups to patients again and managed to identify foods or groups of foods which would reproduce their symptoms, many of which included headache and migraine. He published extensively on this subject in the 1920s and 1930s and, amongst other things, gave details of three trials which studied the relationship between food allergy and migraine. These trials will be described in detail in the chapter on migraine trials (page 119).

The year 1925 was a historic one in the field of allergy and, for those physicians taking a wide view of allergy, an 'infamous one'. The interest in food allergy had just started to grow, particularly in the United States of America. However, in 1925, European and British allergists persuaded their American colleagues to restrict their definition of allergy to those mechanisms which could be explained by the antigen-antibody hypothesis. This, of course made the field extremely 'scientific' — these reactions could be measured accurately in the laboratory and did not depend on the involvement of such nasty and unpredictable factors as actual patients and their own individual observations! The most eminent American immunologist of the day, Arthur F. Coca of Cornell University, fought strongly against this restrictive view, but most of his colleagues in the allergy profession went along with this new orthodoxy. In Rowe's writings he distinguished between immediate and delayed reactions, but he did not discover that what would normally be a delayed reaction could be converted into an immediate one for diagnostic purposes. If a food which is eaten on a regular basis is totally eliminated from the patient's diet for five days and then deliberately fed, symptoms will occur within two or three hours if allergy exists. This delay of two or three hours occurs with foods other than cereals, but the reaction to cereal items tends to be rather slower.

Rinkel's Discovery

The concept of 'masked' food allergy was originally identified by Dr Herbert Rinkel, a well-known allergist practising in Oklahoma City. Rinkel was renowned for being an extremely acute observer of various cause and effect relationships. After he qualified in medicine, he developed a severe nasal allergy called an allergic rhinitis, which is a condition characterized by severe persistent nasal discharge. His medical colleagues skin-tested him for all the well-known inhalant allergies and these tests proved completely negative. He was familiar with Rowe's work on food allergy and suspected he might have such a problem himself. When Rinkel had been a medical student, like many of his colleagues, he had been fairly impecunious. Unlike in British universities, grants are not common in the United States of America and, generally speaking, medical students going through college there have to support themselves or be supported by their parents. Rinkel's father, who was an egg farmer, had supported his son during his medical studentship by sending him a gross of eggs (144) each week and this was the main source of protein for Rinkel and his family. This high ingestion of eggs continued after he qualified and he therefore suspected eggs as a cause of his problem. One afternoon, in an attempt to produce an adverse reaction, he consumed a large quantity of eggs, but to his surprise his nasal symptoms in that afternoon were, if anything, rather improved. Some years later he did the opposite — he abstained from eggs for about five days and then discovered that his nasal discharge improved very considerably. After five days he inadvertently consumed some angel cake (which of course contains egg), at a birthday party. He suddenly collapsed unconscious and his rhinitis returned in dramatic fashion.

Masked food allergy
Rinkel conceived as a result of this experience that he might well have stumbled on something fundamental regarding the basic nature of food allergy. He thus repeated the experiment by re-establishing his consumption of eggs, omitting them again for five days and again repeating the egg ingestion, which caused a recurrence of the symptoms of unconsciousness and nasal discharge. He next extended his observations to a number of his patients and found a similar phenomenon occurring in these patients with a wide variety of different foods and with a wide variety of medical conditions, including migraine. His observations were first published in 1944, where masking was defined in the following way: if a person ingests a particular food each day, he may become allergic to it and yet not suspect this as a cause of his symptoms. It is usual to feel better after a meal than before. In this case the feedings tend to mask the symptoms of the allergic response. Rinkel could not explain his observation which occurred in several thousand patients. Since Rinkel's original work, cases of masked food allergy have been reported in many thousands of patients on many separate occasions. Masked food allergy represents an interesting model of addictive behaviour and is, in my opinion, the major basic mechanism behind the addiction to such apparently diverse items as coffee, tea, sugar, alcoholic beverages and tobacco. This concept can be represented graphically, as shown in Figure 1 (overleaf).

This graph illustrates the results of eating or not eating a masked food allergen in a patient with a single food allergy. Each asterisk represents the feeding of the allergenic food. As can be seen, the second feeding aborts the deterioration of a patient's symptoms as seen after the first feeding. This is followed by an improvement. A similar response is

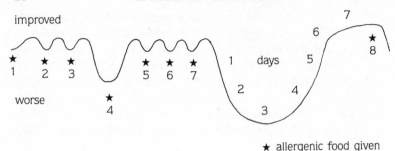

★ allergenic food given

Figure 1

experienced after the third feeding. Because the fourth feeding of the allergenic food is delayed, the patient's response is further down the withdrawal curve and is thus worse. Following this fourth feeding, the patient's condition usually returns to normal. In migraine patients, for example, if this fourth feeding is delayed for too long, a stage is reached when further feeding of the allergenic food is to no avail.

After the seventh feeding, in this example, a patient has been deliberately told to avoid the allergenic food and he or she then exhibits the classic withdrawal phenomenon. This is characterized by a considerable deterioration of symptoms, usually by the evening of the first day. The second and third day tend to be quite severe but are followed by a slow improvement until the sixth day. By the sixth day most patients are symptom-free if under 35 years old. In patients older than 35, the symptoms may take another day or so to clear. Feeding at stage eight represents a deliberate re-feeding and the Rinkel hyperacute response. In this, as illustrated by Rinkel's experience, symptoms return frequently and quite dramatically.

Figure 1 demonstrates how complicated is the relationship between one commonly-eaten food allergen and the symptomatology that it creates. Imagine, therefore, if one is dealing with a patient who has allergies to wheat, corn, milk and yeast, there will be a different curve of symptomatology for each food depending on the frequency at which it is eaten. Any relationship between food and symptoms will in these circumstances become far from obvious. I have emphasized this point to some extent as many physicians believe that if food allergy is present, it will be obvious to all those concerned. It is this simplistic view of the subject which has partly led to its neglect.

This concept of masking is the single most important factor to grasp about migraine. It explains all sorts of observations about migraine which have long been mysterious. It explains for a start why people prone to migraine who fast almost invariably get a migraine — because they are missing their next masking dose of their allergen. Hence it shows why migraine is so common amongst Jewish people on the Day of Atonement. Secondly, it explains why migraine specialists have found from experience that their patients will get less migraine if they have small, frequent meals. They therefore advise patients to eat very regularly. It furthermore reveals why the commonest time to acquire a migraine is on awakening, because at this time of the day it has often been many hours since the migraine sufferer consumed his last dose of allergic food, particularly if it was not present in his evening meal. It explains why many patients have a migraine on a Saturday. On this day they tend to lie in bed for longer than during the week and have breakfast later and therefore there is some delay in the time before they have their next masking feeding. Breakfast, of course, is the meal which tends to be full of common food allergens such as wheat, corn, milk and sugar.

The concept of masking also explains why some foods eaten only on an occasional and intermittent basis have long been known to provoke migraine. Chocolate, cheese, citrus fruits and red wine are thought by most people to be the prime food allergens for migraine, but an inspection of the list of common food allergens discovered by trials which recognize the importance of the masking phenomenon show the commonest food allergens to be wheat, corn, milk, eggs and so forth, which of course are eaten daily in one form or another by most people. A perusal of the results of these trials shows that orange is pretty well the only exception to this rule. It is an intermittently-eaten food in general, but is certainly one of the commonest causes of migraine.

To summarize the position, it is fair to say that a migraine sufferer can contract a migraine either by eating a food consumed only intermittently (usually less than once every five days), in which case they get a reintroduction-type response (Rinkel's hyperacute response), or they can provoke a migraine by *not* eating a food which is consumed at most meals. As the common food allergens discovered in these trials are wheat, corn, milk, eggs, sugar, etc. and these foods are consumed daily by most people, most migraines must be caused by the withdrawal response. People very rarely go for over five days without consuming such items as wheat. In other words, the usual reason for a patient getting a migraine is 'by not consuming a food to which he is allergic'.

Needless to say, these observations which were originally made forty years ago were ignored or misunderstood by the medical profession in general, but a full account of the concept was given in what is now the classic textbook on food allergy. It is entitled *Food Allergy* by Herbert J. Rinkel MD, Dr Theron G. Randolph MD and Michael Zeller MD. It was originally published in 1951 by Charles C. Thomas, but because of the current explosion of interest in this field, it has been republished by The New England Foundation for Allergic and Environmental Diseases of the Alan Mandell Centre for Bio Ecologic Diseases. In this book, the main basic concepts of food allergy are described in great detail.

Food allergies can be basically divided into fixed food allergies and cyclic food allergies. Basically, a fixed food allergy is one which has probably been present since birth and will never go away. In other words, the patient may eat the food extremely rarely but every time he does so he reacts adversely. He may avoid the food for twenty years and then still react strongly to it. These fixed food allergies are comparatively rare and certainly account for less than 5 per cent of all food allergies. For the purpose of definition, a food allergy which disappears within two years of complete avoidance of the food will generally be regarded as a cyclic food allergy and that which has not will be generally thought of as a fixed one. In a cyclic food allergy the degree of reaction is related to the frequency of ingestion. One method of treatment other than desensitization (which is discussed in Chapter 8) is to avoid the food for a period of time, during which tolerance can develop. This time usually varies between two and eight months, but by definition can extend up to two years. Usually, the stronger the symptoms that the food gives, the longer it takes for tolerance to develop. Tolerance can also, in exceptional circumstances, develop within two or three weeks and this is a potent source of problems in elimination diets, which may extend over a period of about five weeks.

Tolerance is, however, a fragile flower and can usually be

maintained only if the patient eats the allergenic food every five days. If the food is consumed more frequently than this, the patient nearly always starts to react to it again. It is, of course, vital that the patient understands this concept. I have seen patients who identify specific food allergies on an exclusion diet. Some months later they may eat the food again by mistake but, having suffered no reaction, they conclude that their original observation was erroneous. Unless forewarned, they may then start to eat the food on a frequent basis, rapidly destroy their tolerance to it and then start to react to it once more. These ideas about the development and subsequent maintenance of tolerance led to the development of what is known as the rotary diversified diet.

The Rotary Diversified Diet
The rotary diversified diet is one of the major concepts and tools in the practice of clinical ecology. Patients with minor allergy problems or with a sensitivity to only two or three foods will rarely need to go on it. Patients who are adequately dealt with by desensitization will not usually need to use it. Patients who have a Candida problem (see Chapter 7) need it less if their Candida is treated. However, all patients, even if they do not go on to a formal rotary diet, are advised to widen the scope of the foods they eat to the maximum extent and to vary their diet as much as is possible. The fundamental principle of the rotary diet is that foods from specific food families are only eaten on one day in every four. A typical rotary diversified diet is as follows on pages 30 and 31.

It will be seen from perusal of this diet that certain principles have been followed in devising it:
(a) only whole foods are included. A food mixture, for example gravy powder, contains: (1) starch — probably corn; (2) modified starch; (3) salt; (4) caramel — probably derived from glucose; (5) soya flour; (6) hydrolyzed vegetable protein; (7) dried yeast; and (8) flavourings. A single product containing such a wide range of items would be inadmissible.
(b) Food families need to be considered in devising a rotary diversified diet. The reason for this is that patients can cross-react to 'relatives' of foods to which they are allergic. Foods from a whole food family are therefore included on the same day but excluded mostly from other days. Another reason for considering food families is that the continual ingestion of

TYPICAL ROTARY DIVERSIFIED DIET

	Day 1	Day 2	Day 3	Day 4
Protein	All red meats and their products: Pork Venison Beef, veal, lamb Milk, yogurt, all cheese	All fish: Tuna, mackerel. Rock salmon Turbot, sole, halibut, flounder Haddock. cod. Perch. Carp Trout, salmon. Sardines, herring	Fowl and eggs: Turkey, goose, duck Chicken, pheasant, guinea hen Eggs	Shellfish: Crab, shrimps, lobster Clams, oysters Snails, squid Scallops
Vegetables	Mushrooms Sweet potatoes Squash, courgettes, pumpkin, cucumber Water chestnuts	Cabbage, broccoli, turnips, radishes, cauliflower, Brussels sprouts, mustard greens, kale Lettuce, artichokes, endive Yams, yuca	Carrots, celery parsnips, parsley All peas and beans, lentils, soya beans, alfalfa sprouts, bean sprouts (legumes) Asparagus, onions, leeks	Spinach, beetroot, Swiss chard Okra Potatoes, tomatoes, eggplant Peppers Corn, bamboo shoots
Fruit	Pineapple Dates Melons Peaches, apricots, nectarines, cherries, plums, prunes	Grapes, raisins Blueberries, cranberries, Bananas Guavas	Strawberries, raspberries, Apples, pears Rhubarb Mangoes Papayas Currants	Oranges, grapefruit, lemons, tangerines Pomegranates Figs Gooseberries Avocado

TYPICAL ROTARY DIVERSIFIED DIET

	Day 1	Day 2	Day 3	Day 4
Seeds and Nuts	Pumpkin seeds Almonds Macadamia nuts	Sunflower seeds Pecans, walnuts	Peanuts, soy nuts Cashews, pistachios Sesame seeds	Filberts, hazelnuts, chestnuts Brazil nuts
Other	Coconut Arrowroot starch Yeast Gelatin	Tapioca Sunflower meal	Peanut butter Sesame meal Buckwheat	Olives Wheat, rye, barley, cornmeal, Popcorn, cane, oats, rice, millet
Sweeteners	Whey, lactose Date sugar	Maple sugar or syrup	Honey	Molasses, malt syrup
Lard and Oils	Almond oil Butter, lard, beef fat Coconut oil	Walnut oil Safflower oil, sunflower oil Any fish oils	Peanut oil, soy oil Chicken fat, turkey fat Sesame oil	Olive oil Corn oil
Herbs and Spices	Nutmeg, mace Black pepper Vanilla bean	Mustard, horseradish Mint, sage, rosemary, basil, marjoram, oregano, thyme Allspice, cloves Cream of tartar	Dill, fennel, caraway, anise, chervil, cumin, coriander Ginger, cardamon, turmeric Garlic, chives	Cinnamon, bay leaf Chilli, pimiento, paprika, cayenne, red pepper
Teas	Rosehips	Blueberry Chamomile, goldenrod Mint	Papaya leaf Senna Parsley. Alfalfa Sarsaparilla	Juniper berry Sassafras Comfrey. Hops

several foods from a family can lead to the development of allergy. If garlic is eaten on Sunday, onions on Monday, asparagus on Tuesday and leeks on Wednesday, then foods are not being truly rotated. One food from this group (which is known as the LILY food family group) is in this case being eaten every day and this can in some cases sensitize people to the whole food group. However, the ingestion of foods from a specific food family does not need to be totally spaced at four-day intervals. Usually two-day intervals will be satisfactory. In other words, with our example from the LILY group, garlic and onions could be eaten on Monday and asparagus and leeks on Wednesday, then garlic and onions again on Friday.

Many people looking at the sample rotary diversified diet will notice in it a large number of foods they have never eaten or even thought of eating in their life. Patients, in my experience, are amazed at how much they enjoy foods they have never considered in the past. An allergy to a food is primarily linked to the frequency of ingestion of that food and so the wider and more varied the diet the better. Obviously, if the patient is not being desensitized to foods, he must omit the foods to which he is allergic from this diet. In the years prior to the development of food desensitization and other developments, for example in connection with intestinal thrush, the rotary diversified diet was the only way of helping the complex multi-allergic patient. It was, however, difficult, if not impossible for some patients such as those who had to attend business lunches most of their working life. I do still encourage patients to vary their diet as much as is reasonably possible but, except in the more severe complex cases, I do not use a full rotary diversified diet. A much more comprehensive account of the rotary diet is given in such books as *Allergies, Your Hidden Enemy* by Dr T. G. Randolph and Dr R. W. Moss and *Coping With Your Allergies* by Natalie Golos and Francis Golos-Golbitz.

The work of Dr Richard Mackarness

In the late 1950s a British doctor, Richard Mackarness, stumbled on to the whole concept of food allergy. One perceptive observer of human behaviour noted, 'when most people stumble over a truly original idea, they smartly pick themselves up, dust themselves down and carry on their way'.

Dr Mackarness was an exception to this rule. In 1958 his book *Eat Fat and Grow Slim* was published. He had before this taken a great interest in obesity and noted that people who lived in primitive circumstances eating primitive foods rarely became obese. He conceived the thought that obesity might result from foods such as cereals and sugars, products which had only comparatively recently been incorporated into the human diet. Whereas fruits, vegetables, meats and fish had been consumed for over 100,000 years, cereals had only been consumed for about 2,000 years and sugar for 300 years. In other words, it was possible that mankind had not had time to adapt to these comparatively new foods. In his book, against the prevailing medical wisdom of the day, he therefore advocated a diet avoiding cereals and sugars, but allowing as much fat, protein, vegetables and other carbohydrates as the patient required. Many patients found this diet very helpful and the book sold in enormous quantity in the United Kingdom. As a result his publishers asked him to do a lecture tour of the United States of America to promote the launch of the book there. At one of these lectures he met a doctor who, having listened to his lecture, said to him, 'I am sure that you are right, but possibly for the wrong reasons. Many of your patients are probably allergic to foods such as cereals and sugars. By warning them off these foods, they are probably becoming better because they are avoiding the common food allergies.' It is, of course, likely that these foods are the common food allergies because mankind has not well adapted to them. This doctor suggested that Dr Mackarness should meet his brother-in-law, who was Dr Theron Randolph. Mackarness responded to this idea with alacrity and, after meeting Dr Randolph, became fascinated by all the ideas that Dr Randolph was able to impart. When Dr Mackarness returned to his practice in Kew he slowly incorporated these new ideas into his day-to-day general practice. Having acquired a fair amount of experience in this field and having become entirely convinced by its validity, he then wrote the now-famous book entitled *Not All in the Mind*, which was initally published in 1976. In 1980 he followed this success with his next book, *Chemical Victims*. With these two books he succeeded in opening up in Great Britain a whole awareness of this subject.

Dr Mackarness would be the first to admit that he had not originated any major new thoughts on this subject but, with his flair for communication honed by his years as medical correspondent of the old *News Chronicle*, he became the greatest living public advocate of the subject. The medical profession as a whole did not like *Not All in the Mind*, partly because the book was aimed primarily at the popular reader and partly because the concepts discussed had not been sustantiated by large-scale clinical trials. However, Mackarness knew that if he wrote the book solely for the medical profession it would have disappeared without trace. At the time he could not substantiate his claims with large-scale clinical trials, as at that time, few had been performed. What Mackarness did know was that he was right and that this new knowledge would eventually change the whole face of medicine. When physicians first saw penicillin dramatically cure meningococcal meningitis, they knew they were witnessing something very significant. They did not need a double-blind controlled clinical trial to prove it to them. Much of the same applies to those physicians who have seen patients with severe chronic symptoms become well within a few days on a low-risk diet.

Spreading the Word

Although the medical profession as a whole was not interested in food and chemical allergy, a small group of doctors, of which I was one, had their curiosity aroused. I arranged to meet Dr Mackarness at Basingstoke General Hospital, where he worked, and talked to him at length and met many of his patients. Very encouraged by all I had seen and heard, I tentatively tried these ideas on my own general practice patients. Immediately I began to see enormous improvements in some of my patients who had had long-term intractable problems. A few other doctors, such as Dr Ronald Finn, a Consultant Physician at Liverpool General Hospital, Drs Radcliffe and Husband who are GPs in Southampton, Dr Kingsley of Osgathorpe in Leicestershire, Dr George Hearn, a Consultant Physician in Birmingham, all became involved very quickly. Within two to three years this number expanded to about nineteen doctors, who in 1979 formed the British Clinical Ecology Group. By January 1982 the number had swelled to over one hundred and the group changed and became the British Society for Clinical Ecology.

Various clinical trials began to be published sustantiating

the claim that food allergy was a very important factor in human diseases, including migraine. Dr Finn in 1978 wrote a paper entitled 'Food Allergy, Fact or Fiction?' This was published in *The Lancet* and the trial he had performed demonstrated that food allergy was the major factor in a series of patients who had, amongst other symptoms, a history of palpitations. The trial was a double-blind trial where patients were fed foods that were suspected to be allergens in situations when they did not know what they were eating. For example, the foods were introduced via a stomach tube. This trial was reported widely in the media and prompted more letters to *The Lancet* than any other trial in the previous few years. In May 1979 Dr Ellen Grant had her trial on migraine and food allergy published in *The Lancet*. This particular trial is described extensively in Chapter 12, as are the findings of Dr Jonathan Brostoff and Dr Jean Monro, who published the results of their trial of migraine and food allergy in *The Lancet* in July 1980.

In November 1982 Dr John Hunter and his colleagues at Addenbrooke's Hospital in Cambridge produced a paper on food intolerance and the Irritable Bowel Syndrome. In this paper, again published in *The Lancet*, they demonstrated that two-thirds of patients with this condition could lose their symptoms if they avoided specific foods to which they had been found sensitive. Like all allergy problems, the foods involved varied quite widely, and a number of double-blind studies were completed. October 1983 saw the publication of Professor Soothill and his colleagues' trial of migraine and food allergy in children. This was a most comprehensive trial and is again discussed later in this book (page 126). In 1984 Dr Pamela Graham and some co-workers at Brighton General Hospital published a paper demonstrating that food allergy was a major cause of eczema in children. This paper was published in *The British Journal of Dermatology*. In September 1984, again in *The Lancet*, Dr Jonathan Brostoff and Dr Jean Monro published yet another study on migraine and food allergy and this is again dealt with in the chapter on the migraine trials. These aforementioned trials are some of the major studies that have been published in the past few years. However, there have been quite a lot of other studies, some of which have been published in the United States of America.

In May 1984 there was a large international meeting of the British and American Societies for Clinical Ecology, held at

Torquay in Devon. At this meeting papers were read by doctors from different parts of the world, reporting studies of food and chemical sensitivity in relation to a number of other diseases, such as hyperactivity in children, recurrent ear infections in children, rheumatoid arthritis and recurrent thrombophlebitis.

The concept that food allergy is an important factor in disease processes has therefore advanced enormously in the past few years. That it is a major factor in quite a number of diseases is slowly becoming accepted. In relation to migraine the evidence now is overwhelming, and I think it can be said that food allergy has been proved to be the major cause of migraine. The detailed evidence for this assertion is contained in Chapter 12.

3.
CHEMICAL ALLERGY AND
ITS HISTORICAL DEVELOPMENT

The idea that food allergy was a major factor in the production of human disease had been considered for many years before anyone conceived that human beings could be individually sensitive to specific chemicals. Now chemical allergy is less commonly involved in the migraine problem than is food allergy, and only in comparatively rare cases is it the whole cause of the problem. However, in countless cases it complicates the food-allergy symptoms, and simply dealing with the food allergies does not entirely solve the problem.

The man who discovered the whole chemical-allergy problem was Dr Theron Randolph, of Chicago, Illinois. Dr Randolph was well-acquainted with the concepts of food allergy which had been promoted by Dr Albert Rowe, Dr Arthur F. Coca and Dr Herbert Rinkel. He had in 1951 written the now historic textbook, *Food Allergy* by Randolph T. G., Rinkel, H. J. and Zeller, M., published by Charles C. Thomas of Springfield, Illinois. He had also been involved in conducting a migraine trial involving 127 patients in 1935, with Dr J. M. Sheldon. This trial is discussed on page 119. Dr Randolph's discovery about chemical allergy was his greatest contribution to medicine. In 1951 he concluded that a number of his patients were reacting to a wide range of petrochemicals in their environment. These petrochemicals were usually present in totally 'non-toxic' levels. Patients could be reacting to either chemicals such as petrol, gas, paint, perfumes, cigarette smoke or formaldehyde, which could be inhaled, or alternatively to chemicals in their food.

The chemicals in food can either be the combination of pesticide and kerosene with which vegetables, especially leafy vegetables, are sprayed, or those such as ethylene gas which are used, for example, to ripen bananas. There is also, of course, the huge range of food colourants, emulsifying agents, preservatives and other food additives, all of which can upset the susceptible individual. Most of these chemicals I have just mentioned share one fact in common, that is that they are derived ultimately from oil and gas deposits, which in turn come about by the decomposition over millions of years of ancient pine forests. This decomposition is aided by enormous pressures and the range of chemicals that are produced are all similar. It is no coincidence that many of these patients with reactions to petrol and gas and so on also react to turpene gas, which is the gas given off by pine trees. The 'blue haze of the rocky mountains' is caused by the gas given off by these mountainous forests of pine trees and it has been known for many years that some patients will react adversely to this gas.

Multiple Fruit Sensitivity

The earliest recognized case of a specific chemical sensitivity was of a man who reported severe headaches whenever he ate apples. This patient discovered one day that when he ate apples from an old orchard that had not been sprayed for many years, he had no adverse effect. Dr Randolph, whose patient this was, later fed him on a double-blind basis several apples, some of which had been sprayed and some not. The patient reliably only reacted to the sprayed items. Suddenly, an explanation was at hand for cases of multiple fruit sensitivity. All the early allergists had noted that many patients claimed they reacted to nearly all fruits, which was surprising as they came from so many dissociated food families. Most of these patients were not, in fact, reacting at all to the fruits themselves, but to the spray residues on them. These sprays permeate the whole fruit and simply peeling the fruit rarely helps. Anyone, therefore, with multiple fruit sensitivities, should obtain a sample of organically-grown fruit to see if the organically-grown item has the same adverse effect as the commercially-produced item. As mentioned earlier, sometimes patients will report multiple vegetable sensitivities and these can turn out also to be chemical susceptibility problems. Leafy vegetables such as cabbage, broccoli, Brussels sprouts, cauliflower, lettuce and spinach are particularly liable to be sprayed and many patients will react to this whole range.

Common Chemical Additives

Chlorinated hydrocarbons are also used to spray the feed of many animals and these chemicals can contaminate the fat, particularly of animals such as beef, lamb and poultry. As the hydrocarbons are mostly located in the fat, removing the fat from these animals can often reduce or eliminate the problem.

Bananas, as mentioned earlier, are normally ripened by exposure to ethylene gas. They are still green when they arrive in Britain as they travel well like this. A few hours' exposure to ethylene gas will make them yellow and a high proportion of patients with hydrocarbon sensitivity react to these bananas, but find non-gassed bananas cause no problem. Some people who apparently react adversely to coffee are in reality not reacting to coffee itself, but to the fact that most coffee is roasted over a gas flame.

Sulphur dioxide is another chemical which can cause problems. Patients are frequently puzzled as to why they react to French-fried potatoes prepared in a restaurant but not to those eaten at home. Almost all restaurants buy pre-cut and packed French-fried potatoes and they are soaked in sulphur dioxide to stop them browning at the edges. Some of my patients who were apparently reacting to corn turned out later to be in reality reacting to sulphur dioxide. I discovered that prior to processing the corn, the corn kernel is soaked in sulphur dioxide solution in order to prevent the corn fermenting.

Cucumbers, apples and green peppers are foods which are frequently coated with paraffin wax to improve their appearance and keep them edible for longer periods of time. This paraffin wax is derived from petroleum and can therefore cause problems similar to those mentioned earlier.

Coming loosely under the category of chemicals in food is the subject of chemicals occurring in our tap water. The most common problem by far is chlorine, which is of course added to tap water in order to curtail the spread of infection. In this context it is very effective, but nevertheless quite a large number of chemically-sensitive patients react adversely to it. It is for this reason that when I place a patient on a low-risk allergy diet, they also use bottled spring water to start with. Most patients with chlorine sensitivity can tolerate tap water which has been boiled for eight minutes. Chlorine is volatile and boiling will normally remove it. There are a range of chlorine filters on the market which many patients find remove enough chlorine for them to tolerate the filtered tap water. Insecticide sprays, if used in large quantities, can permeate down through the soil, washed down by rain water, and therefore can contaminate the underground water tables. Patients who are exquisitely sensitive to these insecticides may find it difficult to find a water supply that they can tolerate, as these insecticides are virtually impossible to remove. These patients sometimes have to end up by drinking spring water collected from underground tables in mountain areas. This is a comparatively rare problem for migraine sufferers in Great Britain, but in the United States of America, where crop spraying is practised on a much larger scale, it is becoming an extremely difficult problem for some patients.

Food colourants have received a lot of publicity, particularly in connection with the causation of symptoms of hyperactivity. The Feingold diet, which eliminates all colourants and other additives from food has been used extensively in dealing with this condition, although in fact it is now known that the additives are only part of the overall problem. Dr Stephen Lockey has spent most of his professional career collecting and collating all the individual symptom complexes that can result from exposure to these chemicals. Headaches and migraine are amongst the symptoms that can be produced by these chemicals in certain susceptible individuals. Obviously items such as coloured ice-creams, confectionery and soft drinks such as colas are well-known to contain such dyes. What surprises many people is that many butters and margarines contain dyes to make them look more yellow.

I have touched only briefly on this subject, which is now becoming a huge subject in itself. It is covered in much greater detail in Dr Theron Randolph's book *Human Ecology and Susceptibility to the Chemical Environment*, which was the first book produced on this subject. There is also extensive coverage in the book *Allergies, Your Hidden Enemy*, again by Dr Theron Randolph, but written in collaboration with R. W. Moss, PhD. Dr Richard Mackarness devoted a whole book to the subject and called it *Chemical Victims*. Many readers may wonder at this point how a physician can possibly sort out all these possibilities, but in fact both the initial history given by the patient and the design of the elimination diet usually enable these matters to be sorted out satisfactorily. When the migraine patient is first interviewed, various pointers can be obtained which may suggest that hydrocarbons may be implicated in the patient's problems. As will be seen in the following chapter, the basic concept is to start the patient on a very simple unpolluted diet and to build up gradually to a fairly normal diet, identifying the problems as the various foods and later chemicals are added selectively back into the diet.

Air Pollution
Inhaled chemical problems can be roughly divided into indoor air pollution and outdoor air pollution and many people may be surprised to learn that indoor air pollution is generally known to be more of a problem. Outdoor air pollution, which is well known because of such phenomena as smog and traffic fumes, is usually only intermittent and often very obvious. The effects of indoor air pollution by contrast are usually more continuous, more hidden, more subtle and more significant. Many hydrocarbon-susceptible patients are aware of the fact that intermittently-presented hydrocarbons such as perfumes, petrol fumes, nail varnish, printer's ink and dry cleaning fluids are able to induce headaches, but they are virtually always ignorant of the fact that their domestic gas or oil is playing a part in their problems. The combustion products of burning these fuels within the confines of the house linger in the house for days, even after the utilities are turned off.

Because of its relative cheapness, natural gas, both for central heating and for cooking, is now present in a very high proportion of British homes. Although gas is more commonly implicated in conditions that have chronic unremitting symptoms, it tends to be less commonly implicated in those migraine sufferers who are perfectly well between their migraine attacks. Many migraine sufferers are, however, permanently fatigued, even between their attacks of migraine or may have a dull background headache almost continuously over and above their migraine symptoms. Such patients can quite often be having problems with pollution within their houses. When this is suspected from the history, we frequently use sublingual or intradermal tests for hydrocarbons in migraine sufferers before tackling possible food allergies. In some patients gas cookers have had to be replaced by electric cookers and gas boilers moved to an outhouse separate from the main building. These expensive manoeuvres are, of course, not carried out until it has been confirmed that the trial of switching off all these utilities and ventilating the house has brought considerable improvement in the patient's health, which has then deteriorated again on turning the utilities back on. Another source of problem for some patients is the vast store of solvent chemicals stored in many houses under the kitchen sink. Paints, varnishes, methylated spirits, cleaning fluids, dry cleaning agents and carpet cleaners all come into this category.

Soft plastics, especially those used to cover clothes returning from the laundry, to wrap food and to wrap items such as pillow cases often trouble some people. The softer, more malleable plastics have a less stable molecular contruction than hard plastics, such as those used in the construction of telephones. The soft plastics, therefore, out-gas more readily and give off a gas called phenol, to which quite a number of patients in my experience react.

Sponge rubber in upholstery, mattresses, cushions and so forth can cause problems with certain individuals. I have not as yet met a patient in whom it actually causes headache, but certainly symptoms like fatigue, restless legs and other insidious problems can be caused by this and many migraine patients report these symptoms in addition to their more classic migraine symptoms.

Cigarette, pipe and cigar smoke are common and usually well-recognized problems in migraine sufferers. Many know long before they attend a clinic that this hydrocarbon contaminant can provoke headaches. The whole subject of cigarette smoking and its relationship to headache and migraine is discussed in greater depth in Chapter 6.

Outdoor air pollution is usually more obvious in its effect. With migraine and headache patients, far and away the most common problem is diesel and petrol fumes. Some patients have observed that long car rides, especially in heavy traffic, almost invariably lead to a headache but have never made the connection that these symptoms are caused by traffic fumes. They sometimes attribute the headache to the stress of driving or, if they are passengers, to the stress of being driven. Diesel fumes are particularly lethal for some patients and if these people find themselves behind diesel lorries or buses they will react adversely, whereas a similar journey in which diesel fumes are not so closely encountered can be accomplished without problem. The back seat of the car attracts more fumes than the front and many people notice they are less affected if they sit in the front seats. A moving car causes a relative vacuum behind it and this can often lead to exhaust fumes entering back windows in quite high concentration unless they are well closed. Most patients with petrol or diesel sensitivity have a history of car sickness as children, which usually improves when they reach their teens, but then becomes replaced by headaches occurring in similar situations. This is an example of alternation, which has already been mentioned in this book. This phenomenon means that a certain specific allergy can cause one set of symptoms at one age and another set of symptoms later in the same patient's life. In practice, all that is happening is that the target organ for the allergen is changing. A high proportion of children who suffer with car sickness are in fact suffering from petrol chemical sensitivity and a history of this problem should always alert the physician to the possibility of a petrochemical problem in later life. Petrochemical sensitivity should be particularly suspected in car sickness when other forms of transport, which involve a fair amount of motion but no contact with hydrocarbons, are found not to cause the same symptoms.

The car sickness of children and the headaches in adults can both be enormously helped in most cases by taking sublingual desensitizing drops of petrol exhaust or synthetic ethanol (See Chapter 9). Many people can then have no problem as long as they take their drops every three or four hours while in the car. A further useful adjunct is a portable negative ionizer which can be plugged into the cigarette lighter on the car dashboard. This helps to keep the level of fumes in the car down to lowish levels. The effect of negative ionizers is very real and they have, for example, been shown in controlled experiments to clear a room of cigarette smoke about thirty times faster than it would normally clear.

4.

THE ELIMINATION DIET

Bearing in mind the concept of masking described earlier, the main problem with the initial part of any dietary procedure for determining specific food allergies is to separate the patient from all the foods to which he is likely to be sensitive, for a period of approximately five to seven days. Obviously, one way of achieving this is a total fast on spring water, but this has several obvious drawbacks, the most obvious one being that most patients cannot or will not do this. In the Western world, the idea of a fast, even for one day, is culturally very difficult to accept. In the Middle East and countries where other religions hold sway, fasting at prescribed periods of the year is often commonplace.

Fasting
Fasting is easier to accomplish on an in-patient basis than an out-patient basis and in the United Kingdom there are as yet few clinical ecology units. Overweight patients tolerate a fast much better than people who are slim. These people universally feel weak by the end of five days' fasting and this weakness often tends to counteract the beneficial effects that should result from their withdrawal from constantly-eaten food allergens. It is for these reasons that, except in the most extreme cases, I personally do not use fasting to separate my patients from the commonly eaten and likely food allergens. On the other hand, I do not favour dietary regimes which just seek to withdraw certain common food allergens from the diet, one or two at a time. There are several reasons for this. Firstly, if a patient is suffering, for example, from eight food allergies and he withdraws two of them from this diet, he may not feel any benefit as he will still be suffering from

the remaining six allergies. As his condition will not have improved, the response when he reintroduces the two suspect foods back into this diet may not be all that obvious. The situation is analogous to what I call the 'eight nails in the shoe' theory. If someone goes to the cobbler with eight nails in his shoe and only two are removed, he will notice little benefit. Even if six are removed, there may be no noticeable benefit. If all eight are removed concurrently, the improvement is dramatic and obvious. The same applies to patients with multiple food allergies. My preference, therefore, is for outpatients with anything but the most severe and complex symptom problems, to go on to a low-risk group of foods for five to seven days, depending on age. In general, children and young adults clear their symptoms in four or five days, whereas middle-aged or elderly people often take six or seven days before they become absolutely symptom-free.

Low-risk foods

The following twelve foods have a low risk of producing allergic reactions: lamb, pears, cod, trout, plaice, carrots, courgettes, avocado pears, runner beans, parsnips, swedes and turnips. The assessment of this risk is based on the experience and conclusions of many allergists working in this field over many years. In addition to having a low allergic potential, these foods also tend to be less commonly contaminated with spray chemicals, etc. than many other foods. For example the brassica family (cabbage, broccoli, Brussels sprouts and cauliflower) is relatively safe to eat, but many patients may react to the insecticide sprays with which the vegetables are almost universally sprayed when obtained from the commercial market. I ask the patient whether he eats any of these items on a fairly regular basis and I exclude any item on this list which is normally eaten more than once every three days (and preferably any item normally eaten more than once every four days). Many children eating school meals, for example, will have carrots virtually every day and in such patients I would not regard carrots as a safe item to use in the original diet. Another criterion for acceptance on this list is relative availability in either fresh or frozen form all year round in Great Britain.

When I treat a young child with a mild to moderately severe migraine problem (particularly one who is not very enthusiastic or well motivated), I would probably utilize all the above twelve foods, unless one was already eaten very frequently. With a reasonably well-motivated adult with a moderate problem, I would probably use lamb, pears, cod, trout, plaice, courgettes and carrots with the same reservations as previously mentioned. Bearing in mind that every extra food eaten in this phase represents a distinct risk of failure, although these foods have a low risk, none of them have no risk at all.

The Elimination Diet

In the first five days, these low-risk foods can be eaten in any quantity. As food allergy is ultimately caused in most patients by eating foods in very high frequency, there is a minor theoretical possibility that a patient may sensitize himself to one of these foods in this period of time. I have put many thousands of patients through diets such as this and I am not convinced I have ever seen this happen as yet. It is certainly much easier and more successful to tell a patient specifically what he may eat in this phase than to give him a long list of food items which he may not eat. It is a major educational feat, for example, to teach a patient which foods contain corn or wheat or yeast or soya beans. These foods should all be prepared 'au naturel'. In other words, no butter must be used on the fish, the lamb must not be basted with a cooking oil, such as corn oil. The fat of the lamb can, however, be utilized for basting and to fry the courgettes. Foods such as pears or carrots can be eaten raw or boiled. The only fluid that is allowed initially is a bottle of spring water, either still or sparkling. There are various types on the market which vary somewhat in taste and have their individual aderents. Basically, any of them are satisfactory for the purposes of this diet. If the patient wishes it, they can prepare a carrot or pear juice by liquidizing these items with the spring water. I allow my patients with migraine to continue to use pure sea salt.

The next extremely important point I make to my patients is that while they are going through this dietary exclusion programme they must completely stop all the medications that they normally take. Virtually all tablets, capsules and liquid medications sold in the Western world contain common food allergens in the form of filling agents, binders or sweeteners. The items most commonly used are corn (or maize starch), lactose, cane and beet sugars, and these foods are all in the most 'likely' category as far as allergy is concerned. In the case of tablets, it is basically solidified corn starch that forms the tablet. Initially, I was mystified as to why corn starch or lactose was used in capsules, but most chemical powders are fine and fly around somewhat unless they are first mixed with the starch prior to going into the capsuling machine. Glucose, cane and beet sugar are commonly used to coat various tablets and in addition there is the whole gamut of colourants used in various tablets, which of course can be a source of trouble in themselves.

Of particular importance in the treatment of migraine is the necessity to come off the contraceptive pill, especially in the evaluation phase. This is partly because of the reasons I have just given and partly because in many patients it is a major cause of migraine in itself. This may be due either to a specific sensitivity to the hormones that the pill contains or through its contribution to the intestinal candidiasis (thrush) problem which will be discussed in detail later. Another major medication to mention in this context is ergotamine tartrate. This is of course, the most specific medication used for migraine sufferers and, although it often helps a lot of patients originally, there is now hard evidence that some patients subsequently become allergic and addicted to it. I have certainly seen a number of patients who never became well until they became withdrawn from this drug. One lady, the wife of a famous inventor, saw a number of clinical ecologists who failed to cure her persistent migraine headaches. Eventually she confessed to one of them that she had never stopped taking her ergotamine tablets, although she had told the other clinical ecologists, that she had. When she did stop taking the tablets her case suddenly became very easy to manage.

Patients on anti-hypertensive medications (for high blood-pressure) also need to stop their tablets. As was noted in Dr Ellen Grant's trial, patients with conventional hypertension who have migraine, usually find that their blood-pressure returns to normal when their food allergies are worked out. Certainly, I have never seen anyone's blood-pressure rise dangerously while on this elimination procedure and most reduce very satisfactorily, despite the absence of the medications. For anyone who is a smoker, it is absolutely essential to stop this habit while going through the elimination diet.

There remain three further pieces of advice of which the patient should be aware:

(1) Sodium bicarbonate solution should be substituted for toothpaste as various components of toothpaste can be absorbed under the tongue and cause problems.

(2) Licking stamps and envelopes can cause problems as the glue contains corn.

(3) A heavy dose of Epsom salts, two or three teaspoons for most adults but maybe one teaspoon for children, should be taken on the morning of the first day of the diet to eliminate existing foods eaten the preceding days prior to the diet.

Of great importance next is the careful selection of an appropriate time to start this procedure. The highly restricted part of the diet only lasts 5½ days, but there is a decreasing degree of restriction for approximately five weeks afterwards. Social engagements like weddings and dinner dances where eating complex food mixtures is virtually compulsory should be avoided, especially in the first three weeks of this procedure. If attendance at such functions is essential, the diet should be postponed until after them, unless the patient is of a particularly stoic and determined personality.

The Process of Elimination

At this point we should recall the description of the masking phenomenon and the withdrawal phase that follows the cessation of eating food allergens. Ninety per cent of patients suffer a migraine starting on the first day of the low-risk diet. Most of these migraines start between 10 a.m. in the morning and 6 p.m. in the evening. Of course some patients with very frequent migraine may well wake up with a migraine on the first day of the diet for the same reasons that they normally wake up with a migraine. The most common time for the migraine to start, however, is early afternoon. By the evening, it is often extremely intense and the evening of the first day and the second day of the diet often see the worst migraine that the patient has had for years. If the patient has fatigue as one of his usual symptoms, then there is often very considerable fatigue at the same time and many patients with bad migraine problems spend the second day of this diet in bed. If the migraine sufferer is prone to depression, then this also can be quite nasty on the second day.

The third day sees some improvement in some patients, especially the younger ones, but many people's migraines continue into the third day, and sometimes even into the fourth. The third day of this elimination diet often sees the onset of aching pains in the main muscle groups, especially the back of the thighs, the buttocks, the lower back and the shoulders. These symptoms are termed 'withdrawal myalgia'. Over fifty per cent of migraine sufferers develop these symptoms in the mid part of the withdrawal phase, although in some cases they can occur as early as the second day or as late as the fourth. These muscle pains usually decrease on Day 5 and disappear on Day 6 or 7. Catarrhal symptoms can often occur, especially on the third day, but they are essentially very short-lived. Day 5 can be quite a good day, especially for young patients, but often Day 6 is the first time that the patient experiences real benefit for his sacrifices. A few patients do not feel really improved until Day 7. Many patients on Days 5, 6 or 7, report considerable feelings of well-being, energy and lack of fatigue and depression and an indefinable sensation that there is no potential headache lurking round the next corner.

The occurrence of severe symptoms in the first three days of the diet, followed by considerable improvement by Day 6 or 7, is excellent proof that food allergy is the basis of the patient's symptoms. By Days 6 or 7, therefore, the patient and his doctor are usually in possession of good evidence that his problems are related to food allergy. At this point, however, it remains to be seen which food allergies are involved. Day 6 of the diet, therefore, is usually a good day for a consultation, to review what has occurred up to that point and for the doctor to instruct his patient in how to broaden his diet. Referring back to Dr Rinkel's observations on masking, it will be recalled that once a food has been omitted from the diet for five days or more the reaction to it becomes sharpened — Rinkel's hyperacute response. The reactions are probably at their most sharp between five and twelve days after the foods are first omitted, but they are usually fairly obvious for a few weeks, after which time some degree of tolerance begins to develop in many people.

The Reintroduction Programme
There are many ways in which foods can be brought back into the diet. In deciding on a reintroduction programme several factors should be borne in mind.

1. After 5½ days on a very limited diet, the patient will very much welcome a broadening of their diet and so the addition of a few foods to which they are not likely to react will usually be a helpful idea. Foods such as broccoli, runner beans, beef, rice, melon, tomatoes, pineapple, lettuce, apples, grapes and chicken all come into this category. They can be reintroduced at a rate of one per meal, as long as the meals are separated by about five to six hours. If there is going to be a reaction to these foods it will normally occur within this period of time. The most common time for a reaction to occur is approximately two to three hours after the food is ingested.

2. The next principle that should be observed is that foods from the same food family should not be introduced within four days of each other. If a patient reacts to one citrus fruit today, it is possible, because of cross allergenicity within a group, that if another citrus fruit is introduced two days later the reaction to this food will be masked by the reaction to the first citrus fruit.

3. Clearly, there is no point in testing a food mixture. The observation that a piece of cake causes the patient to react is pretty valueless as it does not tell the investigator whether the reaction is to the eggs, the cornflour, the cane sugar or the beet sugar and so forth. It follows, therefore, that the main basic contributors to the diet, such as wheat, corn, rye, oats, malt, cane sugar, beet sugar, yeast, soya beans, eggs, potatoes and milk should all be tested in pure form. If the patient reacts to pure yeast powder, it can be assumed that all products containing yeast will cause a similar reaction.

4. The cereals, especially wheat, corn, oats and rye, are all very slowly absorbed and will rarely react as quickly as most other foods. I accordingly arrange to test these foods in pure form for a period of two days each. The cereal is eaten at every meal in those two days and most commonly the reaction starts some time on the second day. In some people, however, it will start on the first day and they can obviously abandon the test at this point.

In assessing reactions to food a number of further points should be considered:

1. In a patient with, for example, migraines, non-migrainous headaches, fatigue and depression, one food may cause some symptoms, another food other symptoms. If the food induces fatigue or depression or a headache, it should be elminated, even if the symptoms are reasonably bearable. The easiest patient to deal with is the patient who is feeling better than he has felt for years and any variation from this well-being should be very easy to spot.

2. Reactions to foods come in all shapes and sizes and intensities like everything else in life. Severe reactions are obvious to the patient, who is usually amazed at the dramatic transformation from feeling particularly well to particularly ill. Moderate reactions are usually also fairly obvious to spot, but mild reactions can pose a problem. The patient may not be sure whether the onset of a mild headache is related to a food, some emotional crisis, prolonged reading or some other factor. Usually emotional upsets in themselves do not produce a headache and only act as a triggering factor in someone already suffering from food allergies. The way in which this in-doubt situation can be resolved is of course by re-testing. Hence the two rules that govern this situation are: (a) if in doubt about a food, leave it out; and (b) never re-test a food in less than five days from the original test. If one re-tests before five days have elapsed, the reaction may not be noticed because of the masking phenomenon.

3. If a patient suffers from a reaction and, for example, has migraine and fatigue, then clearly while he is suffering from these symptoms, further testing is impossible. All food testing is entirely dependent on the patient being essentially symptom-free before the test starts. If the patient waits for the symptoms to resolve spontaneously, he may well find the reaction will last one to three days, during which time he will be unable to continue his testing routine.

An effective medication for these reactions, which will not interfere with the general allergy assessment, is a mixture of bicarbonates. The mixture normally advocated is: two level teaspoons of sodium bicarbonate, plus one level teaspoon of potassium bicarbonate, which should be dissolved in about ¼ pint (140ml) water (this should be spring water until tap water has been tested). The water should be as hot as the patient can drink in one gulp. The potassium bicarbonate is often difficult to obtain from retail chemists, but it can be obtained by the chemist from certain wholesalers. This mixture is relatively unpleasant to take for the patient, but it is usually remarkably helpful. If works on one hand by giving most patients a bowel movement and eliminating the offending food, and on the other hand by correcting the relative acidosis caused by the food reaction. The acidosis which follows food reactions and which can be measured causes many of the symptoms, and partially correcting it by administering a large dose of alkali produces considerable improvement. One or two doses of this alkaline mixture with plenty of fluid by mouth will normally reduce the reaction time by about fifty per cent. Once the symptoms have abated, further testing can commence. Single item foods are therefore tested one at a time. When a food has been passed as safe, it can be eaten from then on. After a reasonable range of standard meats, fish, fruit and vegetables have been tested, then the main dietary constituents such as wheat, corn, milk, cane suger, beet sugar, yeast, eggs, potatoes and soya can be introduced.

It will be noticed that cane and beet sugar are tested separately, although chemically they are both sucrose. These sugars, however, come from totally different parts of the plant kingdom and the biological contaminants produced by their differing biological ancestry is primarily responsible for the differences in their allergic potential. After all these foods have been tried, the main chemical additives should be tested one at a time. Most delicatessens sell pure crystalline monosodium glutamate, saccharine and various standard food colourants. Other food additives such as bleaching agents and preservatives can be tested by eating foods which contain these items and which have otherwise been found to be compatible. For example, if the patient can tolerate wholemeal bread but reacts to white bread it is likely that he is reacting to the added chemicals, which are usually the bleaching agents or the anti-staling agents. These chemicals are used in a wide range of manufactured foods.

The yellow-golden lining on tins of food is also worth testing. This lining is called a phenolic resin and its purpose is to prevent the tin oxidizing and blanching the food it contains. This test can be accomplised in a patient who is not allergic to carrots (an uncommon allergy) by testing some tinned carrots. It is, incidentally, important not to use one of the brands containing sugar, particularly if the patient is known to be sensitive to sugar. There are a number of other chemicals which are often worth testing, but it must be emphasized that reactions to chemical additives in foods are far less common in the average migraine sufferer than allergies to the main foods, such as wheat, corn, milk, cane and beet sugar, soya and yeast.

5.

THE MANAGEMENT OF FOOD AND CHEMICAL ALLERGY

It is perhaps appropriate at this stage to discuss how the principles I have just discussed in the last two chapters work out in real life. The cases I have chosen have been selected because they are ordinary and represent the daily run-of-the-mill cases as opposed to the occasional, unusual, fascinating, perhaps bizarre cases which tend to stick in the mind of physicians doing this work.

Case Histories

Mr R. A., aged 54, came to see me several years ago. He told me that he had suffered from several migraines every month since the age of 18, in other words for 36 years. In addition he complained of persistent and debilitating lethargy and his weight was always inclined to be high, usually around 14st 9lb. His blood-pressure was slightly high at 145/85. He regularly took two drugs, Migraleave and Dixarit, to relieve his attacks.

He was put on a low-risk diet (see Chapter 4) and had a severe withdrawal migraine on the first day. On Days 2-6 of the withdrawal period he had a great deal of muscle pain (withdrawal myalgia) and also fatigue. The myalgia and fatigue disappeared by Day 6, by which time his weight had dropped by 1 stone and his blood-pressure had dropped to 120/90. On this sixth day he felt remarkably well. In the course of re-eating specific foods in the next few weeks he was found to have strong reactions to corn, potatoes, chocolate, instant coffee and white bread (but not wholemeal bread). When seen several months later, his weight had stablized at 13st 10lb and his blood-pressure at 125/80. He told me that, apart from having absolutely no migraines at all, he was feeling extremely well, better than he could ever recall. He felt very bright and alive and very energetic in the evenings in contradistinction to his situation prior to treatment. I saw him again at yearly intervals for the next two or three years and this improvement was maintained in all forms. Whereas his reactions to potatoes and corn were straight food allergies, his reaction to instant coffee as opposed to pure coffee was clearly a chemical one, that is a response to the anti-staling agents used to preserve instant coffee. The reaction to white bread was also presumably due to the anti-staling agents used.

Mrs I. G. aged 54, had suffered from migraine for the preceding twenty years and in addition had had mild headaches almost daily in this period of time. Her migraines occurred on average twice a month and the only other symptom she had was lethargy. She had been treated with Dixarit, which had decreased the intensity of her headaches, but their frequency had increased. In the withdrawal phase she had a migraine lasting for the first two days, followed by a mild headache for the next two days. By the sixth day she was feeling well. In the next few weeks she had severe reactions to wheat and corn but otherwise felt very well. By avoiding wheat and corn she remained completely free of migraine throughout all her follow-up visits extending over the next few months.

An example of a patient with multiple food sensitivities was a Mrs S. S., aged 68, who had a history of migraine extending over forty years. Her migraines occurred on an average of three attacks per month, but she had headaches to some extent literally every day of her life. The migraines consisted of headaches plus nausea and severe visual phenomena. She also gave a history of palpitations and swelling of her ankles. She normally took Cafergot tablets for her migraines. On the restricted diet, in her case lamb and pears, she had a classic withdrawal response with severe migraine occurring for the first three days. By the sixth day she was remarkably improved. In the next couple of months she showed severe reactions to wheat, corn, oats, rye, artichokes, chicory, lime, cod, plaice, sardines, grapes, gooseberries, currants, coriander, leeks, cabbage, broccoli, turnips, raw carrots, parsnips, green beans, lentils, peas, peanuts, soya beans, peppers, pineapple, almonds, apricots, peaches, plums, tomatoes, chocolate and coffee in all forms, including even the smell of coffee. She subsequently found in the succeeding months that there was a tendency for her to develop allergies to foods which on first testing had appeared to be satisfactory. Accordingly, she was put on a four-day rotation of foods according to families and subsequently remained extremely well. One year later she told me that she was still feeling splendid, had no headaches at all or migraines, was feeling very energetic and felt that her life had completely changed. Although the list of foods to be avoided was rather daunting, she had worked out a very extensive diet of less commonly-eaten foods which she thoroughly enjoyed. This lady's problem had been solved in the days before my discovery of the intradermal technique of desensitization. If she same to see me nowadays, she would have been extensively desensitized to the main foods in this list.

An example of a rather off-beat food-allergy problem occurred with Mr G. B., aged 22. This young man presented me with a history of weekly migraines occurring in the preceding three years with gradually increasing frequency. He had no other symptoms whatsoever. On the low-risk diet he had a severe migraine starting at midday on the first day of the diet and lasting for the first two days. By the third day he was feeling reasonably well, but there was still a degree of muscle aches and pains which had started on the first day. By Day 4 he was symptom-free. We then started introducing foods back into his diet, but this period was remarkable because of the total lack of reaction. I had formed an impression from talking to him that he was likely to be allergic to coffee, as he was fairly addicted to this. To my surprise, he reacted neither to ordinary coffee beans nor to instant coffee. After he had been through the whole reintroduction of foods period, there was still no reaction at all. However, when he had his first cup of coffee at work, he had a reaction within half an hour. On reading the label of the coffee supplied at his work, he realized it was a French coffee containing chicory. The reaction to chicory was confirmed when he deliberately took some chicory essence one week later and suffered perhaps the severest migraine he had ever had. Various foods closely related to chicory were carefully tested without producing any reaction, and we came to the conclusion at the end of his investigation that his only reaction was to chicory. He, of course, had been having chicory in all the coffee he drank at work and in retrospect it was obvious that his migraines started within a week or two of taking up the job. I happened to see him two years after he had been treated and he had told me that since that day he had had absolutely no migraines, nor even a trace of headache. This particular case emphasizes the individuality of this problem. This young man is the only patient I have ever seen out of well over a thousand who has had a reaction only to chicory. It is a rare item to be allergic to in any case and for it to be the basis of the whole problem is unique.

A more typical type of patient was Mrs J. C., aged 33, who consulted me earlier this year with a 3½-year history of migraines. The usual frequency was about two migraines per month, each of which lasted two days. One of the migraines was almost inevitably on the first day of her period. In addition to the migraines she noticed quite a lot of fatigue and some bloating of her abdomen after food. On the low-risk diet of about six foods she had a standard withdrawal response and by about Day 7 or 8 felt extremely well, with far more energy than she had been used to for years. She subsequently reacted to wheat, yeast, onions, coffee, oranges and, rather strangely, turkey and lentils. Her worst reaction by far was the one to wheat, where she had a severe migraine developing on the second day of the test. Her reaction, for example, to onions just involved some visual disturbance. She was subsequently tested intradermaly to get her neutralizing points to the above foods, except for turkey which we decided she could avoid. She received her neutralizing levels by subcutaneous injection, which she administered to herself on alternative days. She is currently eating all the foods to which she is sensitive without any adverse effect.

This case is probably the most representative of the ones we see, with an average of about six or seven food sensitivities. Almost all of our patients we now treat with neutralization therapy to enable them to eat the foods to which they are sensitive. The details of this technique are set out in Chapter 8.

Another case in which chemical sensitivity complicated the picture was Mrs J. C., aged 39, who reported a history of very severe migraines since the age of six. With her migraines she suffered nausea, vomiting and frequent visual problems. She had a minimum of five attacks per month and spent an average of seven or eight days per month in bed. Before she attended the clinic, she knew that chocolate, onion and Stilton cheese upset her, but these were clearly not the only causes of her problem. She had found most drugs relatively ineffective.

On the low-risk diet she was struck by a very severe migraine, starting on the first day, but was well by the morning of the third day. On the six day she felt extremely well, in fact better than for many years. Her eyes looked bright and she felt very energetic. On re-eating specific foods, she found that she reacted to orange, rice, coffee, matured cheeses and the whole of the LILY group of foods, that is onion, garlic, asparagus, chives and leeks. She reacted to many dried fruits but not the undried versions, and this suggested an allergy to sulphur and/or methyl bromide, which are both used in the fumigation process. Other ingested chemicals to which she reacted included monosodium glutamate and preservatives in general. While avoiding these ingested items, she only had symptoms as a result of contact with fumes from marker pens or diesel lorries. She took steps to avoid these contacts and in the subsequent five years she became virtually migraine-free.

Mrs S. C., aged 37, had a history of approximately six migraines a month for the preceding 2½ years. Over the same period of time she had suffered from severe bouts of depression and almost continuous lethargy. Her weight was 9st 13lb. She regularly took Valium 2 mg three times a day, Imipramine (an anti-depressant) 25 mg three times a day and the sleeping tablet Mogadon. She was placed on the low-risk allergy diet and all her medications were discontinued. A severe migraine developed on the first day of this diet and continued on the second day. By the third day the migraine had subsided, but was replaced by strong generalized muscle pains (myalgia), starting on the third day and easing out by Day 6. By this sixth day she was quite well and her mind felt much clearer. She had lost 8½lb in 5½ days. On reintroducing foods back into her diet, she had a severe reaction to wheat, which proved to be her only food allergy.

She would occasionally suffer a minor headache when in contact with petrochemicals, such as on long journeys by car through heavy traffic. She found that if she took sodium cromoglycate in its nasal and inhaled forms before such contacts there would be no problems. On her last follow-up visit she reported no migraine, no headache, no depression and no lethargy. She felt totally cured and all her friends had noticed a marked change in her demeanour. She also felt that she was able to achieve much more in a day than she had been able to do at any time in the preceding years.

A patient with more troublesome chemical problems was Mrs B. W., aged 27, who had a history of severe migraines extending over the previous two years. Her attacks had averaged about four per month and she told me that in these attacks she had headache, vomiting and pins and needles on the right side of her body. She would take DF118, either by tablet or injection, for her attacks. On the low-risk diet she had a moderate headache on the second and third day, but no other symptoms. In the reintroduction phase she reacted only to corn and corn products.

She did, however, notice a number of reactions to inhaled chemicals which were constant and reproducible. These included cigarette smoke, certain perfumes, petrol and diesel fumes, ether meth and phenol (the hospital disinfectant smell). She had had, for example, headache reactions whenever she visited a friend in hospital. She found that sodium cromoglycate protected her from these problems, though nowadays we would have probably used specific neutralization therapy. At her three-monthly follow-up visit she reported that she was entirely well.

In 1976, a few months after I first became interested in this subject, I was consulted by a Mrs Amelia Nathan-Hill, who was and still is a committee member of the British Migraine Association. This lady had probably the most severe problem with migraine that I have ever heard of or encountered. She had had severe migraines for well over thirty years. Every morning she would wake up with a headache and this would develop into a severe migraine about three times every week. She also complained of abdominal pain, persistent mouth ulcers and severe fatigue.

Her medical problems were so intense that she found that she was spending more time in bed than not, and she travelled extensively throughout the world to various clinics and doctors in the hope of finding a cure for her problems. When these clinics failed to help her she tried various fringe practitioners, faith healers and even a witch-doctor. After I had seen her she went on to a hypoallergenic diet of lamb and avocado pears. On this diet she had a severe withdrawal response in the first few days, but by the sixth day she had lost her headaches for the first time. She subsequently reacted to an enormous number of foods — well over forty — and this work-out procedure took her over three months, due to the frequent reactions encountered. Remaining on her 'good foods' she became totally migraine- and headache-free. Interestingly, her fatigue, mouth ulcers and minor patches of eczema also cleared up completely. Her only remaining symptoms were feeling of heaviness and muzziness in her head first thing in the morning and she still suffered from her colitis problems to a minor degree. Later it was discovered that she had a sensitivity to gas and when the gas was removed from her house, there was another quantum improvement in her general symptomatology. Later, when the intestinal thrush concept was discovered, she was treated for this and became virtually symptom-free on all counts.

For the first few years after she first came to see me she had to avoid a huge number of foods and rotate the good foods so that she did not develop further sensitivities. Later, when we had the facilities, we desensitized her to a large number of foods and she became able to eat these foods without adverse effect. She was so impressed with the treatment that when she became well, she decided to set up a charitable organization to encourage and collate research in this field. This organization became known as 'Action Against Allergy' and, with her driving force behind it, it rapidly became very well-known and successful. Currently it has about 1200 members. It activities include lectures and symposia and it also has an extensive library of books relating to this subject. Having easy access to these books, many of which are published in the United States of America, has helped to spread information on this subject extensively in this country.

I have used Amelia's full name in this respect, as she has already written extensively about her condition and her response to this treatment in her book entitled, *Against The Unexpected Enemy*. This is a moving account from a patient's point of view of her struggles against her medical problems and her eventual victory over them.

These case histories illustrate the enormous variability of the migraine problem. Many cases are very straightforward and need only to go through a simple elimination diet and avoid the incriminated foods. Others are much more complicated and need consideration of their chemical problems and possibly extensive desensitization.

6.

THE ROLE OF ALCOHOL, SMOKING, THE PILL AND ERGOTAMINE IN MIGRAINE

1. Alcohol

Very large numbers of migraine sufferers know that alcohol, often specific alcoholic beverages, will invariably precipitate their migraine. Some, for example, will note that red wine may precipitate their problems and others may notice the same problems with other certain specific spirits or wines. Some migraneurs will observe that all alcoholic beverages will cause their problems.

In the late 1940s, Dr Theron Randolph made the considerable intuitive leap in realizing that reactions to alcoholic beverages were caused by reactions to the constituents of these beverages and not to the alcohol itself. What made the reactions to these beverages so obvious is the rapid absorption of their constituents. Everyone is familiar with the very rapidly observable effect of, for example, four double Scotches consumed in quick succession. The main constituent of Scotch whisky is wheat which when consumed normally (i.e. in the form of bread) takes many hours to absorb in any quantity. In the form of Scotch whisky, it is absorbed in a few minutes. Part of the reason for this rapid absorption is that whereas food is normally only absorbed in the intestines, alcohol is absorbed throughout the whole intestinal tract, starting from the mouth, going through the stomach and duodenum into the intestines. Dr Randolph coined the phrase that reactions to alcoholic beverages represent 'food allergy in a jet-propelled vehicle'.

Most of the main alcoholic beverages are derived from foods such as wheat, corn, cane sugar, yeast, grapes, potatoes and so forth. As I have stated elsewhere in this book, these items represent the more common food allergens. Remembering the concept of masking, it is obvious that to a wheat-allergic patient a dose of an alcoholic beverage containing wheat will have a quicker masking effect than wheat eaten conventionally because of the rapid absorbative effect. Hence, if allergy to wheat can lead to addiction to wheat, addiction to Scotch whisky will follow if the patient is not careful. Alcoholism has been termed the acme of food allergy and there is no doubt in my mind, having dealt with a number of alcoholics, that this is true. Sometimes, however, the rapidity of the absorption of the alcoholic beverage is such that it 'breaks through the masking process' and can give the patient a direct reaction to the food rather than a masking effect.

Conversely, if the alcoholic beverage contains a substance, for example grapes or a resin or a preserving chemical which is not regularly present in the patient's diet, then he may well have an unmasked hyperacute reaction, made even more acute by the rapidity of absorption.

Alcoholism and Food Allergy

The fact that alcoholism and food allergy are inextricably interwoven is of course important in managing migraine patients who are addicted to alcohol. In most cases these patients are allergic/addicted to the common constituents of alcoholic beverages, such as cereals, sugar and yeast, and this allergy/addiction can only be eradicated if the foodstuff is concurrently removed from both the patient's diet and from his drinking habits. Because of the widespread ignorance of this concept, alcoholics usually continue to eat the foods to which they are allergic while manfully trying to avoid them in the form of alcoholic beverages. The dried-out alcoholic is therefore depriving himself of his quickest and most effective 'masking shot'. Most feel tense or depressed or headachy and the desire for alcohol often remains extremely strong for many years.

It follows from this that some alcoholics in whom specific allergies have been identified can, as long as they modify their drinking habits, consume certain alcoholic beverages without suffering a reaction. This ingestion, though, has to be done with some caution as there is a chance that the patient will develop a sensitivity to another food if he has a predilection to food sensitivities in any case. If this new food is consumed freqently in this very potent form, i.e. alcohol, it is quite possible that new sensitivities will arise, and so such consumption should be limited to occasional social events. The exception to all of this is, of course, the patient who has a yeast sensitivity, as yeast is present in all alcoholic beverages. As yet, there has been no large published series in which the interrelationship of alcohol and food allergy has been investigated. There have, however, been numerous individual case reports, particularly from Dr Theron Randolph, Dr Marshall Mandell and Dr Richard Mackarness, and their observations have all supported this view. I have seen many remarkable results myself adopting this approach and one patient particularly sticks in my mind.

I was consulted in 1978 by Mr W. K., aged 44, a dried-out alcoholic. The beverage to which he had been addicted had been vodka, and since ceasing to drink it he had remained extremely tense, necessitating the ingestion of approximately 60 mg of Valium each day. He also suffered from numerous headaches and he told me he felt he was on the verge of returning to his drinking habits. After six days on a low-risk allergy diet, he felt immensely improved and discovered he had no need to take Valium any longer. He reintroduced foods to his diet in a similar way to that described in Chapter 4. He was fine until he tried potato (a major constituent of most vodkas) and the ingestion of this food reproduced all his old symptoms. At the time of this reaction, I had immense difficulty in persuading him to keep on his diet and to keep off a vodka binge. He managed to keep to my advice and the reaction wore off in a couple of days. Subsequently, avoiding potatoes, he had no need to take any more Valium, had no tension, no headaches and no desire to start drinking again.

The law does not require that the contents of alcoholic beverages to be stated on the bottle and in general they are allowed to remain a trade secret. However, as a result of discussions with representatives of some major alcohol manufacturers, it is possible to put together a rough guide to the content of the major alcoholic beverages obtainable in this country. Most of the information presented below relates predominantly to products from the Distillers Corporation, who are the major suppliers of alcoholic beverages in this country. Vodkas, for example, can be made from a very wide range of foods and the vodka cited in this example is made by Smirnoff. Much of the information which is presented here was subsequently verified by patients with known food sensitivities who have managed to observe which alcoholic beverages they can tolerate and which they cannot. There follows a breakdown of the alcoholic beverages which are most commonly consumed in the United Kingdom.

It must be added that wines may contain a number of chemicals which are not mentioned in this list. The cheaper wines, particularly those imported in bulk, will normally have chemicals added to them to stop them deteriorating while travelling. As most travellers know, cheap wines do not travel well in the normal course of events and preserving chemicals have to be added to maintain them in good condition. Reaction

Always present = ✓ / Sometimes present = 0	Corn	Wheat, Barley, Rye	Oats	Rice	Potatoes	Grapes	Plum	Citrus	Cherry	Apples	Hops	Juniper	Cinnamon	Mint	Miscellaneous Herbs	Cactus	Beet Sugar	Cane Sugar
Blended Scotch Whisky	✓	✓															0	0
Malt Scotch Whisky	0	✓															0	0
Canadian Blended Whisky	✓	✓				✓	✓	0									0	✓
Irish Whisky		✓	✓															0
Blended Irish Whisky		✓	✓	✓		✓	✓	0									0	0
Gin (Grain)	✓	✓	0	0				✓				✓	0	0	✓		0	0
Gin (Cane) High & Dry												✓	✓	✓	✓			✓
Vodka				0													✓	✓
Jamaican Rum																		✓
Tequila																✓		✓
Beer	✓	✓	0	✓							✓							
Grape Brandy	0					✓											0	0
Cordials and Liqueurs	✓	✓	0	0	0	✓	✓	✓	✓	✓			✓	✓	✓		✓	✓
Grape Wine	0					✓											✓	✓
Sherry	✓					✓											✓	✓
Champagne						✓											✓	
Cider	✓									✓							✓	✓
Vermouth	0	0	0			✓											✓	✓
Cognac						✓											0	0
Cherry Brandy	0								✓								0	0

Please note that yeast occurs in all alcoholic beverages.

to these chemicals is extremely prevalent and accounts I think for the common observation that cheap wine can cause a nasty hangover and headache, whereas more expensive wine does not. The severe hangover which certain patients may experience with certain alcoholic beverages is usually due in my opinion to specific food sensitivities occurring in those particular beverages. A more comprehensive review of this subject is given by Dr Theron G. Randolph in the book entitled *Clinical Ecology*, published in 1976 by Charles C. Thomas. The review is Chapter 31, pages 321-33.

2. Smoking

Smoking, and particularly cigarette smoking, has a major effect on the production of migraine in many patients.

In Dr Ellen Grant's trial, published in May 1979 in *The Lancet* and mentioned in Chapter 12 of this book, a pilot study was performed prior to the main study to look briefly at the effect of smoking, the contraceptive pill and ergotamine tartrate as single entities. A group of thirty smokers were advised to stop smoking, to avoid cheese, chocolate, citrus fruits, alcohol and other people's cigarette smoke. Very rapidly 53 per cent of this group became headache-free. Only 13 per cent of a group of non-smokers who followed this same dietary advice became headache-free. The 40 per cent difference between these two groups was presumably due to the absence of smoking in the cigarette smokers. The effects of smoking in this trial were perhaps most graphically illustrated by the following table:

Total number of headaches per month for 30 patients, before stopping smoking and after stopping smoking with simple dietary advice

Smokers (30)	Number of Days With		
	Migraine	Headaches	Daily Headaches
Before	169	380	12
After	16	71	1

Smokers (30)	Number of Patients With	
	Hypertension	Headache-free
Before	5	0
After	1	16 (53%)

In the past the role of smoking in migraine has been underestimated because surveys of migraine sufferers have shown that the incidence of smoking in migraneurs is the same or marginally less than in the population in general. In 1975, a Migraine Trust survey of 989 Polly Peck factory workers found that the incidence of smoking was the same amongst those with or without migraine. There is, however, evidence that many migraine sufferers have an abnormal sensitivity to cigarette smoke, which causes them to desist from smoking as soon as they first try it. This may be the factor which leads to a lower than expected incidence of cigarette smoking amongst migraneurs. In those migraine patients who smoke, the evidence is that the smoking habit starts many years before the migraines become apparent, and by the time they do the correlation between smoking and migraine is far from obvious. In Dr Grant's trial, the men had been smoking a daily average of 22 cigarettes for 23 years, but the average length of migraine history was only eight years. Thus, on average these patients had smoked cigarettes for 15 years before the problem materialized.

It is interesting to speculate what it is about cigaretttes or other forms of smoking that causes these problems with migraine sufferers. As with all items that are ingested or inhaled on a frequent basis, it is possible that human beings can become sensitized and as allergies seem to be linked with frequent exposure, it is not surprising that some people can become sensitive to something they are exposed to maybe twenty to forty times a day. Often after testing, patients appear to have reacted to the whole of the Solanaceae food family. This food family contains tobacco, potatoes, tomatoes, peppers, aubergine (eggplant), etc. The cigarette smoking has probably sensitized these patients to all of these foods. Tobacco may cross-react and therefore cross-mask with these other food items. A very frequent observation is that cigarette smokers find it much easier to give up smoking on a low-risk food allergy diet than they would normally do on a normal diet. One reason for this may be the absence of cross-reacting and cross-masking to foods from the same food family.

Of great interest is the relationship of sugars to the smoking problem. Most physicians working in this field have noted a high incidence of sugar allergy/addiction in cigarette smokers. Some of the addiction to tobacco appears to be related to sugar and to illustrate this, one has only to cite the well-known phenomenon in which people who are trying to give up smoking transfer their affections to other forms of sugar such as confectionery.

American blended cigarettes are manufactured from a blend of flue-cured, burley and oriental tobaccos. Sugars, liquorice and coca are added in a process which is known as casing. Further 'top-dressing' flavours are usually applied. The precise recipes for the casing and flavours are closely guarded by the manufacturers. Therefore, in the case of American blended cigarettes, the allergy/addiction may be predominantly due to the sugars. In these cases the person who ceases smoking but continues with a diet still containing sugar keeps his sugar addiction going, but is deliberately avoiding the twenty or more masking effects that his cigarette smoking normally affords him. Also, as cigarette smoke is inhaled, the masking occurs very much more rapidly than when sugar is ingested. In these circumstances, it is no wonder that the cigarette smoker finds it hard to give up his smoking. If, however, he goes on to a hypoallergenic diet at the same time, he will of course avoid concurrently both inhaled and ingested sugar and in my experience by about Day 5 on such a diet, most patients find that their addiction to cigaretttes has pretty well ceased.

In the case of cigarettes originating in the United Kingdom, the situation is rather different. The cigarettes are usually manufactured from flue-cured tobacco without any additives. The flue-cured tobacco typically contains approximately 15-20 per cent natural sugar. This sugar is a dextrose-type sugar but unlike the dextrose in our diet it is not manufactured from corn and therefore it is unlikely (as far as we know at present) to cross-react with other sugars in our diet. In the case of cigars originating in the United Kingdom, there are no additives, but many cigars from other sources, for example the USA, have added materials such as sugar.

Pipe tobacco in the United Kingdom is made from both flue-cured and burley tobaccos. Sugars are usually added in the form of glucose, fructose or sucrose. Rum and other flavouring materials are also frequently added. In the USA the additives are similar.

Therefore, to summarize the relationship of smoking to migraine, one can say: (a) a clinial trial has demonstrated that the cessation of smoking with minor dietary advice will frequently lead to the cessation of migraines; (b) cigarettes, cigars and pipe tobacco may all contain items which can cross-react and cross-mask with other items in the diet; (c) it is frequently observed that for these reasons it is much easier to stop cigarette smoking on a low-risk food allergy diet than it is while on a normal diet containing such items as potatoes, tomatoes, peppers and the various sugars.

3. Oral Contraceptive Steroids

I deliberately use this heading to emphasize that oral contraceptives *are* steroids, which is a fact that many physicians lose sight of very easily. Most practising GPs are well aware of the fact that the onset of migraine and headache can frequently coincide with the original prescription of the contraceptive pill. In such patients, two or three types of contraceptive pill are tried and, if they all have the same effect, the patient usually discontinues the medication of her own volition. However, there are some patients who may have a much subtler long-term adverse response. Dr Grant's trial also studied the effects of giving up oral contraceptives. Like the smokers, these migraine sufferers were given the usual minor dietary advice. After giving up oral contraceptives as well as avoiding chocolate, cheese, citrus fruits and alcohol, 33 per cent of the oral contraceptive users became free of headaches. As 13 per cent was the success rate in people who followed the dietary advice without smoking or taking the Pill, the difference of 20 per cent looks as if it may be related to the contraceptive pill.

How the Pill exerts this adverse effect is not completely known. All contraceptives are steroids (cortisone-like chemicals) and have an effect on the immune system and it is, of course, the immune system that is intimately involved with the whole problem of migraine. It may be that the minor suppressing effect of the Pill on this system causes it to go completely off balance, making it easier for food sensitivities to occur. However, in my view, it is more likely that its main effect could be through the promotion of chronic intestinal thrush. In Chapter 13, The Roots of Allergy, I will talk about work which suggests that intestinal thrush is the root cause of many food allergies. What is known for certain is that by suppressing the immune system steroids like the contraceptive pill encourage the proliferation of intestinal thrush, which can lead to the development of more food sensitivities.

4. Ergotamine Tartrate

Ergotamine tartrate is the most frequently used specific remedy for migraine and it is often quite effective. It is, however, a very potent drug and all the literature about it emphasizes that it should be taken in limited dosage. The manufacturer's own data sheets warn that ergotamine tartrate should not be taken for prevention, not more than four tablets should be taken in a single attack and not more than six tablets taken in one week. Many migraine sufferers ignore this advice. Also in these data sheets, it is categorically stated that indiscriminate use of this product may precipitate upon discontinuation of the drug, *withdrawal symptoms amongst which headaches feature predominently.*

The clinical impression amongst many physicians, including myself, is that in some patients ergotamine initially exerts a wholly beneficial influence and patients become very dependent on it. Later, the patient can become sensitive to it and, although it continues to have some beneficial effects, it also becomes part of the problem. Such patients can have enormous difficulty when they try to stop taking the drug. I have had a number of patients who, on reintroducing ergotamine tartrate having gone without it for a week, will get a reaction just like that which occurs when a food allergen is reintroduced. If such patients do not stop their ergotamine, their migraines persist despite help with dietary manipulations.

In Dr Grant's trial, however, the advice to stop ergotamine, combined with the usual simple dietary advice, only resulted in 13 per cent of the patients becoming headache-free, which is the same as the 13 per cent who improved on the dietary advice alone. I have no doubt, however, that erogtamine tartrate can be a migraine precipitant. From Dr Grant's trial, however, it appeas to be less of a problem in this respect than smoking or the contraceptive pill.

7.

THE INTESTINAL THRUSH FACTOR

In October 1981 I attended the 15th Advanced Seminar of the Society for Clinical Ecology held at Callaway Gardens in Atlanta, Georgia. On the programme of this seminar was a lecture by Dr Orion Truss concerning the relationship of thrush *(Candida albicans)* to human disease. Like most of the delegates to that conference, I was familiar with the whole subject of food, chemical and inhalant allergy and its relationship to many human diseases. Also, like these delegates, I was aware that the diligent application of these ideas would solve many chronic disease problems, but that there would be an obstinate minority of patients who would not respond.

What Dr Truss said in effect was that patients could react adversely to the microflora in their own digestive tracts. This concept did not initially strike me forcibly, but I was rather intrigued to observe that most of the out-of-hours discussion at this conference centred around this subject. I met many physicians who excitedly told me how using his concept, they had managed to help dramatically many patients whose problems had been totally resistant to previous efforts. Amongst conditions that were mentioned was migraine. As can be seen in Chapter 12, the highest success rate was 93 per cent and this was in children where allergy problems are less complex and the Candida/thrush situation plays a smaller role. In adults the highest success rate quoted has been 85 per cent. What then is happening to the remaining 15 per cent? I now know that many of these non-responders have problems related to the thrush phenomenon. Dr William Crook has written a book called *The Yeast Connection,* which is entirely about this whole phenomenon. In it he states, 'Since I first learned of the relationship of *Candida albicans* to human disease, my life and practice has changed dramatically. I can hardly wait to get to my office each day because I know I will be seeing people I can help'. I feel very much the same way myself and to analyse my feelings logically I would say that, using standard clinical ecologic techniques, one has a substantial success rate but that one tends to remember the failures, though, more than the successes because they are the patients who, because of their problems, inevitably take up most of the time. With many of these patients also being helped, my professional life is becoming more satisfactory than before.

Candida Albicans

Dr Truss, who practises in Birmingham, Alabama, made the discovery in the mid 1970s that chronic intestinal thrush is a potent factor in the causation of human illness. This discovery will, I am sure, rank as one of the greatest medical discoveries of this century once the implications of it are realized by the medical profession in general. It has been well known for many years by all doctors that the intestinal tract of most human beings is extensively colonized by various bacteria and yeasts and that figuring prominently in this situation is a yeast-like organism called *Candida albicans*. This is known to most laymen as thrush. To most physicicans and laymen thrush is considered to be an organism which can cause a white vaginal discharge in adult females and white plaques in the mouths of babies. It is also sometimes implicated in various minor skin disorders.

The presence of Candida in the intestines has been well recognized for many years, but it has generally up to now been regarded as a pretty innocent bystander. It has been known, for example, to flare up and cause minor bowel problems after courses of antibiotics. In some cases of recurring vaginitis, the intestinal thrush has been treated with courses of an antibiotic medication called *Nystatin* to reduce the intestinal reservoir, thereby hoping to eliminate further vaginal infection. Dr Orion Truss's contribution was that he came to realize that Candida had a much greater role in the causation of human disease than had been previously suspected. As Candida proliferates, it can change in form from the normal yeast-like form to a mycelial fungal form. It has been well known for many years that Candida can exist in either of these two states. The yeast-like state is non-invasive and probably harmless. The fungal form produces long root-like mycelia which can penetrate the mucous membrane of the intestine. This penetration can lead to 'leaky mucous membranes' in the digestive tract and allow incompletely digested dietary proteins etc. to come into direct contact with the immune system, which is basically not designed to deal with such high-molecular-weight items. Hence, patients who have a chronic overgrowth of *Candida albicans* and a high percentage of the mycelial form of this frequently show a wide variety of food and environmental allergies. A few years ago an article in *The Lancet*, abstracted later in the Society for Clinical Ecology Newsletter, covered a controlled study indicating that patients with food or skin allergies had leaky mucous membranes which could admit many more protein molecules than was normal. Patients with multiple food and chemical sensitivities thus became that way because antibodies were formed to the antigenic proteins in food, pollens and even, and importantly, their own normal microbiological flora. In addition to causing a leaky intestinal mucous membrane, it has now been convincingly demonstrated (see Chapter 13), that Candida produces a specific toxin called Candida toxin, which seems to have the ability to weaken the whole immune system in general and make it less able to cope with allergy problems.

Whole books have been devoted to this subject. One such book is *The Missing Diagnosis* by Dr Orion Truss and another is *The Yeast Connection* by Dr William Crook. The best evidence that intestinal candidiasis is a major cause of food allergy is the observation by many physicians that the vigorous treatment of intestinal candidiasis seems to lead to considerable improvement in patients with food allergy. Furthermore, by reducing the loads on the immune system, further food sensitivities seem less likely to occur. Most clinical ecologists have reported that the treatment of intestinal candidiasis where appropriate has led to considerable improvement in the general management of the condition. This applies particularly in the difficult, complex, refractory-type case. In these cases in particular, the minor food sensitivities seem to disappear quickly and neutralization treatment of the major allergies tends to be more successful in that the neutralization levels appear remain more stable. As a result of my clinical experience in treating many patients, I feel that this diagram represents from a practical point of view the relationship of Candida to the symptoms of migraine.

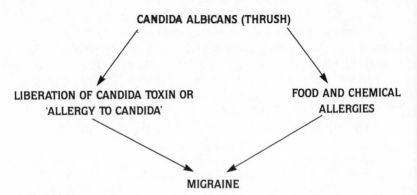

Diagnosis

The diagnosis that chronic intestinal candidiasis is important is based primarily on the whole clinical picture, established by taking a history from the patient. There is as yet no blood test which will indicate categorically when Candida is an important underlying cause and when it is not. Ultimately, if the physician is encouraged by the clinical picture he will treat a patient. If the patient responds to the treatment, then the diagnosis is confirmed. Thus, a therapeutic trial, which is well known and respected in other areas of medicine, is the only ultimate test. The clinical picture consists of the existence of: (a) predisposing factors, and (b) clinical symptoms.

Factors which predispose to chronic intestinal candidiasis are:

(1) Recurrent or prolonged treatment with antibiotics. All physicians know that antibiotics stir up intestinal candidiasis, but what they are not so universally aware of is the long-term adverse effects that can thereby accrue. The worst antibiotics in this respect are the broad-spectrum antibiotics such as tetracycline. These antibiotics kill a lot of the more innocent micro-organisms in the digestive tract and thereby encourage *Candida albicans*. The worse single example of this is the current frequent practice of treating teenage acne with courses of tetracycline, often extending over several years. I have seen many patients who have had severe problems after such treatment.

(2) Prolonged use of the contraceptive pill. The pill is an immunosuppressive drug and, as Dr Ellen Grant frequently points out, is a steroid — in other words a cortisone-like drug.

As a result Dr Grant always insists on calling oral contraceptives 'oral contraceptive steroids' to emphasize this point. I think she is right because both doctors and patients frequently lose sight of the fact that the patients are actually taking a steroid. Steroids work basically by suppressing the immune system and anything that suppresses the immune system will allow Candida to proliferate more easily.

(3) Prolonged treatment with cortisone or cortisone-derived drugs for any particular reason.

(4) Multiple pregnancies.

(5) An environment containing a high proportion of mould. There is a fascinating interaction between environmental moulds and *Candida albicans*. It has been particularly fascinating for me since I have been aware of the Candida problem to notice that people with severe candidiasis frequently are particularly bad in the mould season of the year, which in the United Kingdom is August, September and early October. These patients tend to be particularly bad on damp, humid days in August and September when the mould count is clearly high. They will be frequently improved dramatically by desensitization to moulds in addition to their Candida treatment. If these patients live in damp houses with a lot of mould on the walls in the bathroom and in the kitchen, steps should be taken to eradicate these moulds as far as possible. Various techniques have been described in relation to this, but they are beyond the scope of this book.

(6) A history of high consumption of sugar in the past. A lot of Candida sufferers crave sugar in any form and in fact it is one of the diagnostic features of the condition. Frequently the craving amounts to a total addiction.

(7) Ingestion of large quantities of yeast products.

It will be noticed that all these predisposing factors, with the exception of environmental moulds, are items which have steadily increased with advancing civilization.

Yeast started to be used by human beings about 8,000 years ago, but only in a small way. Nowadays yeast products occur prolifically in our diet. Yeast is present in all leavened breads, all alcoholic beverages, all cheeses, mushrooms and most fruit juices. The consumption of sugar, which was totally unknown in Europe prior to the sixteenth century, has increased dramatically throughout this century and the consumption of sugar per head of the population has increased over thirty-fold since the beginning of the twentieth century.

Antibiotics have been with us to some extent since 1942, but most of the broad-spectrum antibiotics did not arrive until the mid and late 1940s. Cortisone and the contraceptive pill began to be used in the 1950s. All these items are now being used in progressively increasing quantities from year to year.

Symptoms Suggestive of Intestinal Candidiasis

Candida can lead to an enormous range of symptom manifestations and the symptoms can vary enormously from one patient to another. The commonest and most characteristic symptoms are:

(a) Bloating and gaseous distention of the abdomen.
(b) Chronic rectal irritation.
(c) Repeated or chronic thrush vaginitis.
(d) Recurrent bouts of what is frequently called cystitis. This frequently is in fact cystourethritis. Bacteriological cultures of the urine are negative and there is no direct specific evidence of Candida albicans because the infection is deep in the cells of the urethra and bladder.
(e) Recurring depression, irritability, inability to concentrate and problems with memory.
(f) Chronic nervous indigestion-type symptoms, especially in the upper part of the digestive tract. These symptoms are often erronously diagnosed as hiatus hernia.
(g) Chronic constipation, sometimes alternating with diarrhoea.
(h) Recurring fungal-type rashes in different parts of the body.

Virtually nobody has all of these symptoms and of course they can be the result of processes other than Candida. The presence of a fair number of these symptoms is highly suggestive of the problem, but what absolutely clinches the diagnosis is that these symptoms are aggravated by factors which classically aggravate thrush — in other words, they are often made worse by courses of antibiotics or large consumptions of sugar and yeast.

Treatment

The treatment of chronic intestinal candidiasis is usually a fairly prolonged business and at times can be quite difficult. We currently use one or a combination of the following three methods: (1) Nystatin plus diet; (2) Nizoral plus diet; and (3) Lactobacillus acidophilus plus diet. Diet is extremely important in the treatment of candidiasis and it probably is about half of the total treatment in itself. Intestinal thrush is quite resistant to treatment and so on one hand we have to starve the thrush out by depriving it of what it thrives on, and on the other hand attack it with various medications. The diet advocated by various doctors varies somewhat in the severity of the restriction advised. The absolutely ideal diet to combat thrush would contain no carbohydrates at all, but this would be dangerous to the general health of the patient. The diet therefore represents a reasonable compromise between the needs of the patient nutritionally and the speed with which the ultimate result needs to be attained. The degree of restriction also of course depends to some extent on the severity of the individual patient's Candida problem.

All physicians who have treated this problem are agreed that sugar is the most important single item to be avoided. This food is the most easily available source of nutrition for Candida, which proliferates rapidly when it can obtain it. All sugars should be restricted and this includes cane sugar, beet sugar, glucose, powdered fructose, honey and maple syrup. I allow most of my patients to eat some fruit which of course does contain fructose, but I ask them to restrict the total quantity within reason.

Yeast is also very important and therefore items containing yeast should at least initially be restricted. These items include bread, alcohol in all forms, cheeses in all forms, vinegar, mushrooms and citrus fruit juices. Fruit juices that are home-squeezed are allowed but commercial fruit juices have yeast added to stabilize them and this is never, in my experience, mentioned on the label. Bread which is prepared without using yeast, that is soda bread, (made with sodium bicarbonate) is also acceptable and there are recipes available for people to make their own bread. An increasing number of bakeries now seem to be making this bread, which is quite palatable.

Dried fruits should be mostly avoided, as the mould present on them can stimulate the Candida yeast in the intestines. Some doctors limit the total quantities of carbohydrate to about 60-100 grams a day. I do not do this, except in severe cases and for most of my patients I just advise them to take a reasonably low amount of carbohydrate.

Nystatin

The most effective medication to reduce the colonies of *Candida albicans* is Nystatin. Nystatin has been used by doctors for over thirty years and has an enviable safety record. This safety record is partly due to the fact that, except at very high dosage, it is not absorbed at all from the alimentary canal. In other words, it does not reach the blood-stream, but remains inside the digestive tract, where it does all its work, killing the yeast germs situated therein. An illustration of the safety of this medication comes from the cancer institutes in America, where some children have been found to be suffering from virulent intestinal candidiasis as a result of the cytotoxic drugs that they have been given. In these children doses of 100 tablets a day or more of Nystatin have been used to treat these conditions and have been found to be perfectly well tolerated. Nystatin is arguably the safest medication in the British pharmacopoeia.

Most of the doctors I know use pure Nystatin powder rather than Nystatin tablets, which are obtainable at the chemist. I use pure Nystatin powder because: (1) it is much cheaper than the tablets which, when the full dosage is obtained, can be prohibitively expensive; (2) the Candida organisms colonize the whole digestive tract from the mouth to the rectum and, of course, tablets which are swallowed will not treat the organisms in the mouth or the oesophagus; (3) the tablets contain food colourings and other chemicals and filling agents, such as corn starch. These can contribute to the patient's allergy problems or compromise an elimination diet.

The Nystatin powder must be stored in a refrigerator, but not in the freezer compartment. The most usual dosage regime is to start taking Nystatin at a dosage of half a level teaspoon per day. The teaspoon should be a 5 ml plastic measuring teaspoon. The half-teaspoon dosage is placed into any cold drink that does not contain sugar or yeast and stirred well until it dissolves. This total daily dose of half a teaspoon is taken in four equal doses and spread at roughly equal intervals throughout the day. Ideally the powder should be taken an hour or two before food is ingested. After a week, if there are no problems, the dosage is increased to three-quarters of a teaspoon. In most cases, the dose is therafter increased by one-quarter of a teaspoon every week until a total dosage of two teaspoons a day is attained. The problems that can occur can take various guises. Sometimes there is a marked aggravation of the symptoms that are actually being treated. On other occasions one can see the development of symptoms such as headache, fatigue, depression and flu-like features. Interestingly, it appears that these symptoms are not a direct reaction to Nystatin, as they decrease or stop within four or five days if the Nystatin level is just reduced. Futhermore, they can occur with any form of anti-Candida treatment. Although the precise mechanism of the production of these symptoms is not fully understood, it is virtually certain that they are a reaction to the sudden absorption of large quantities of dead Candida germs. With the germs being killed there may well be a large liberation of Candida toxins. In other words, the Candida germs are being successfully destroyed and the body is having an 'allergic-like' reaction to the dead Cadida, or a reaction to the success of the treatment. This sort of reaction is termed a Herxheimer reaction after Dr Herxheimer who, many years ago, described a similar response when patients were being successfully treated for syphilis. In this case they were reacting to the dead spirochaetes (syphilis germs).

Any patients experiencing this sort of reaction can be sure that they have a Candida problem, as people without the Candida problem have no trouble at all in taking any dosage of Nystatin. These Herxheimer responses are for most people temporary set-backs in the treatment. The patient merely reduces the dose of Nystatin for a few days to approximately half of the dosage which produced the reaction. The symptoms usually clear in four days and then the dosage can be gradually increased again. In most cases the next time the patient reaches the dosage level that caused problems there is no recurrence of symptoms.

There are some patients, it must be said, who have a great deal of trouble getting on at all with Nystatin. These are usually patients with severe chemical allergies and they may have to use a totally non-chemical approach, such as Lactobacillus acidophilus.

Ketoconazole

Another chemical approach to this subject is the use of the drug Ketoconazole, which is sold in the United Kingdom under the trade name of Nizoral. There are definitely some patients who seem to tolerate this drug much better than they do Nystatin. I tend to use the drug only in comparatively short courses, as its safety with prolonged adminstration has not really been demonstrated. Even using the drug for short courses, there is a slight (about 1 in 10,000) risk of hepatitis and blood tests for liver function need to be performed at regular intervals if this drug is to be used for anything over a few weeks. Ketoconazole, unlike Nystatin, is absorbed from the digestive tract and is carried by the blood circulation to the rest of the body. Consequently, it will treat Candida germs in the skin, vagina and in any other tissues. I have a general impression tht it seems to kill Candida a little less dramatically and more smoothly than Nystatin and that patients taking it are often less likely to have a Herxheimer reaction. It also has the advantage that the 200 mg twice-daily dosage is quite a lot cheaper than Nystatin when it is used in full dosage. To summarise therefore, Nizoral is a useful second-string medication for this problem. Personally I have never had any major problem prescribing it, but it does not have as exceptional a safety record as Nystatin.

Lactobacillus acidophilus

A non-chemical approach to Candida is the use of *Lactobacillus acidophilus*. This is a micro-organism which normally resides in the digestive tract of all people. On average, an adult will have approximately 3½lb of various micro-organisms present in the lower small intestine and colon. *Lactobacillus acidophilus* figures prominently in this population of micro-organisms and is wholly beneficial. There are over 200 known strains of *Lactobacillus acidophilus*. Only one strain has marked anti-bacterial activity and this has been marketed in the United States of America as Megadophilus and in the United Kingdom as Superdophilus. Superdophilus has a guaranteed one billion live *Lactobacillus acidophilus* cells per gram and all in all is a much more potent and effective product than some of the other *Lactobacillus acidophilus* products present on the market. Superdophilus is retailed in 2½ oz and 4½ oz amber jars and should be kept refrigerated and never exposed to temperatures above 80°F (26.7°C).

Lactobacillus acidophilus exerts its beneficial influence by actively competing for space on the mucous membranes of the digestive tract with colonies of *Candida albicans*. It is also thought to have a specific antagonistic effect on the *Candida albicans*. In general, I find *Lactobacillus acidophilus* works far slower and less dramatically than Nystatin or Nizoral. Its main use therefore is in instances when the more potent drugs cannot be tolerated. It also aids beneficial recolonization of the gut after Candida has been largely eliminated.

Oleic Acid and Biotin
Another couple of products which are non-chemical and also helpful in combating candidiasis are oleic acid and biotin. Oleic acid is found in cold-pressed olive oil and linseed oil. It acts by inhibiting the fungal form of *Candida albicans* and encouraging the yeast form. It is normally taken, for example, as cold-pressed olive oil in a dosage of two teaspoons three times a day.

It has been discovered that the conversion from the yeast form of *Candida albicans* to the mycelial form is partly dependent upon a deficiency of biotin. It is thought that biotin when given orally can prevent the conversion of Candida to its mycelial form. It is usually taken in a dosage of 500 mcg two times daily.

Desensitization
Another treatment used by many allergists treating the problem is vaccination using extracts of *Candida albicans*. I use *Candida albicans* extract in varying strengths in the same ways as I use food or inhalent extracts to desensitize patients to foods or inhalants (as described in Chapter 9). Neutralizing doses of *Candida albicans* can be dramatically effective in helping the patient, especially in the short term. The response is sometimes so dramatic that it totally convinces the patient that his problems are related to *Candida albicans*. The disadvantage of this treatment is that the neutralizing level of *Candida albicans* has an awkward habit of changing rather rapidly, necessitating retesting at frequent intervals. Sometimes desensitization with TCE, which is a mixture of trichophyton, *Candida albicans* and epidermophyton, can be

even more successful. Trichophyton and epidermophyton are two other fungal micro-organisms found in the digestive tract and they cause problems very much in the same way as *Candida albicans.*

Case Histories

To illustrate the way in which intestinal thrush interacts with food and chemical allergy and further complicates the picture, we can cite three case histories of people with migraine in whom this concept has appeared to be very important.

Mrs B. S., aged 47, had a history of migraines occurring once per week for many years. She also complained of severe constant fatigue, pains in her chest and a runny nose which troubled her throughout most of the year. In traffic fumes she noted that her concentration was very poor, suggesting to me that she might have a sensitivity to vehicle exhaust fumes. As a result of this piece of information we tested her reaction to household gas and, as it was positive on skin test, the gas in her house was turned off during the elimination diet.

On the hypoallergenic diet she had a severe migraine occurring on Days 2 and 5, but rather surprisingly not on Days 3 and 4, which I would have expected. However, by Day 6 she felt really well.

On introducing foods back into her diet she reacted to wheat, rye, cane sugar, rice, eggs, turkey, onion, orange, monosodium glutamate, potatoes, melon, pineapple and tap water. Some of these foods produced diarrhoea, some fatigue and some migraine. Between the reactions she felt very well indeed. At the end of the elimination diet she was desensitized to all the main foods to which she was sensitive, and she then underwent tests to obtain neutralizing levels so that she could protect herself against petrol fumes with the appropriate sublingual drops. As she still had her runny nose problem, neutralizing levels were determined for the common perennial inhaled allergies, such as house dust, house dust mite and so forth. When these were administered to her by injection her rhinitis virtually disappeared. Taking her desensitizing injections for foods and inhalants, she continued to be pretty well. However, as she had several minor symptoms suggestive of intestinal candidiasis, and particularly as she had a distinct chemical problem, we decided to treat her with Nystatin in high dosage and put her on a sugar-free, yeast-free diet.

When she was seen four months after the treatment had been instituted, she reported that there had been a further quantum improvement in her condition since Nystatin had been introduced into her treatment. There was now absolutely no migraine and the fatigue and pains in her chest had completely disappeared. Her runny nose problem was very much improved, but present slightly. Most significantly, she had noticed that inhaled chemicals no longer appeared to affect her at all. Although she had moved the gas boiler from the interior of her house, she was still in contact with gas at the place where she worked and this gas had noticeably stopped affecting her. She had also found that she no longer needed her desensitizing drops for her car journeys.

Dr Orion Truss has often stated his view that chemical reactivity is just part of the Candida problem and improves greatly when the Candida is treated. Case histories like this, of course, support his view.

Mrs F. V. was a married lady, aged 34, who consulted me early in 1984. She gave me a story of severe persistent headaches, which had been present for the preceding four years. Even worse, there was quite distinct depression, for which she had seen several psychiatrists and for which she had been taking antidepressants, such as Ativan. Other symptoms were persistent fatigue, puffiness of her ankles and fingers, minor bouts of fast-beating heart, bouts of sweating at night, distinct problems with weight and a chronic cystitis problem for the preceding year.

After listening to her history, I gained the impression that most of her symptoms were directly due to food allergy and put her on a low-risk diet of about six foods. She had a classic withdrawal response on the second day with severe migraine and depression, but by Day 6 she was very substantially better. As is common with many patients as they go through this elimination diet, after six days her eyes looked clearer, her skin looked far more healthy, and she appeared much more relaxed. Clearly substantial changes had occurred in those six days.

On reintroducing foods to her diet, she had reactions to a number of foods, but her biggest reaction by far was to wheat. Within a day she had severe headache and very marked depressive symptomatology. She had slower but obvious reactions to corn, oats, potatoes and rice. Virtually all her symptoms had cleared, apart from the chronic cystitis. At this point we instituted desensitization therapy to cope with her food allergies, but at the same time put her on a sugar-free diet combined with increasing doses of pure Nystatin powder. We elected to use the anti-Candida approach, partly because of her cystitis, which was highly suggestive of chronic intestinal candidiasis, and partly because she had several food allergies and we felt that they could well be secondary to the Candida problem in the first place. She took increasing doses of Nystatin and built up her level in several weeks to the full daily dosage of two teaspoons. After a few weeks her cystitis disappeared and she became very well in every respect. She found she was eating the foods to which she was sensitive very satisfactorily while taking her subcutaneous desensitizing injections. After about three months of taking Nystatin in full dosage, we were able to tail off the treatment and she continued to remain perfectly well.

Mrs G. H., aged 63, consulted me primarily about her migraines and daily headaches, but she also mentioned that she also suffered from sinus troubles, almost continuous sore throats, a burning sensation around her eyelids, chronic cystitis and thrush vaginitis and distinct weight problems. On further questioning, she told me that she suffered from a bloated abdomen after eating, and rectal irritation. These symptoms, taken in conjunction with the other ones, pretty well confirmed the presence of intestinal thrush. Even more evidence was supplied by her statement that antibodics made all these thrush-like symptoms very much worse. Antibiotics, as mentioned earlier, are notorious for 'aggravating' thrush.

Mrs G. H. improved considerably on the hypoallergenic diet, but she became confused with the food testing, as she had a lot of reactions. We therefore elected to test all her usual foods by intradermal provocation testing and treat her suspected intestinal thrush with increasing doses of Nystatin powder and a sugar-free and yeast-free diet. In addition, as there was evidence in her history that her sinus problems were due to inhaled allergies, such as house dust, these items were also tested for and neutralized. In the course of taking her history, it had also emerged that hydrocarbons such as perfumes, petrol fumes, paint fumes and certain glues made her eye irritation very bad. Provocative skin testing revealed strong reactions to these items and neutralizing sublingual drops were given to protect her against contact with them. After skin testing her to thirty foods and then restricting her diet to these thirty foods, she was given neutralizing injections for the foods which were positive. On this regime she had a marked improvement. In the meantime Nystatin was being given in increasing doses, eventually up to 2½ teaspoons daily.

At her two-month follow-up visit, she reported that her migraines and daily headaches had gone entirely. She occasionally had a mild-to-dull headache, the sore throats had gone and the sinusitis had virtually ceased. The sublingual desensitizing drops were protecting her against the cigarette smoke, perfumes and so on. The symptoms of cystitis and vaginitis had greatly improved, but were still present to some extent. We anticipate that with further anti-Candida treatment, possibly changing to Nizoral, we will completely eradicate the local genito-urinary problem.

These multiply-sensitive patients frequently have a strong history of intestinal candidiasis and from experience it is possible to say that the inhaled chemical problems in the case of Mrs G. H. are almost certainly secondary to the Candida problem. As stated earlier in this chapter, we have had many cases in which the chemical problems have markedly improved after anti-Candida treatment has been completed.

To sum up, Candida appears to be a very important factor in the causation of migraine, sometimes acting directly and sometimes acting through the intermediary of food or chemical sensitivities. When Candida is working in a direct fashion, the only way of dealing with the migraine is by dealing with the Candida itself. When it has its effects through the intermediary of food or chemical allergy, it is still worth treating, as otherwise the patient may well develop further food or chemical allergies or change his/her neutralizing levels to these allergies. The main problem with Candida is knowing when it is important and when it is not. The other potential problems are in the length of treatment needed and, sometimes, the Herxheimer responses. The advantages of treatment for Candida, as we have seen, is that in certain situations it can change a patient's intractable medical problems in a way that is wondrous to behold.

8.

NEUTRALIZATION AND DESENSITIZATION TO FOODS

In late 1977 I had been working in the field of food allergy for about two years and I had a very large number of patients with migraine and other complaints related to food allergy, who had been satisfactorily 'diagnosed' and who knew that as long as they avoided certain specific foods, they would be free of their symptoms. The problem was, however, that the implicated foods were very often common items such as wheat, corn, sugars, milk, egg, yeast and so forth. As can be imagined, a patient with three of these allergies would find it very difficult to attend a cocktail party, a wedding reception, business dinner or almost any other major social occasion without either appearing to be an obsessional food faddist or, alternatively, resigning themselves to the inevitable migraine which would afflict them a few hours after the occasion. Certainly it would be relatively easy for people catering for themselves to keep to a restricted diet, especially if they rarely ate out in restaurants and did not attend many social functions. In contrast, a company executive, might be expected to entertain clients to business lunches almost every day of his working life and he would be unlikely to impress his clients if he had to cross-question the waiter about the content of the menu. Indeed, his 'obsessional' behaviour might even turn his business associates against him.

Taking as an example corn, one of the commonest allergies involved in migraine, I will give some idea as to how difficult it is to avoid this one food. Corn is present in corn oil, which is used widely for cooking. It is almost always present in any product that contains vegetable oil, for example margarine. Corn is found in any item containing cornflour, such as cakes, biscuits, tinned soups, gravies, sauces and custard. It is usually present in any product containing edible starch, which usually means corn starch.

This is present in countless tinned foods, such as baked beans, ravioli and so forth. Corn is present in virtually all products containing glucose. Glucose is nearly always made from corn in this country and the Americans call glucose corn sugar or corn syrup. Glucose is, of course, present in colas, lemonade, and other fizzy drinks, tonic water, bitter lemon, most squashes and virtually every soft drink on the market. The only soft drinks which do not contain glucose are some of the slimline versions of the items already mentioned and pure fruit juices. Corn is also present in many alcoholic beverages and I refer the reader to page 65 where the main constituent of alcoholic beverages are listed.

Being comparatively 'non-tacky' form of sugar, corn is also found in a wide range of confectionery and chocolates. It is also one of the major components of most breakfast cereals. People are often surprised when I tell them that it is used as a filling agent in some cheap coffees, and corn starch is the main filling agent and binder in most tablets and capsules on the British pharmaceutical market. Glucose, in addition, is a common constituent of many liquid medications, such as antibiotics and cough linctuses.

Therefore, this one food can in itself be incredibly difficult to avoid and, in practice, most people with a corn allergy are not completely successful and suffer a return of symptoms whenever they slip up. One patient of mine, who suffered from a corn allergy and who had to entertain guests for lunch at restaurants daily, ended up with as many migraines after he was told about his corn allergy as he did before he knew about it. However, he told me that whenever he was away from the office he could remain migraine-free. In his case, a simple de-sensitization to corn completely changed his condition and his migraines ceased promptly.

Accordingly in late 1977, I became aware of the intense need for a technique to desensitize my patients to such difficult-to-avoid foods. I had heard that various American clinics were then using a technique to desensitize people to foods and when I attended the advanced seminar for clinical ecology in San Francisco in October 1977, I took the opportunity of visiting Dr Phyllis Saiffer's clinic in Berkeley, California. I was highly impressed at the technique and the enthusiatic reactions from patients to whom I talked. I later spent time at Dr Miller's clinic in Mobil, Alabama, and gathered all the literature I could obtain on the subject. Having purchased a range of reagents and other necessary equipment, I started tentatively to try the new technique on patients who had well-defined food allergies. To my delight, most reported that within a few days they could eat the foods to which they were sensitive without adverse effect.

The doctor credited with the discovery of this technique was Dr H. Carlton Lee of Kansas, Missouri. Dr Lee made the startling observation that, whereas certain concentrations of food when injected intradermally (between the layers of the skin) could induce symptoms in a patient, another concentration of exactly the same foodstuff could relieve these same symptoms and in fact could protect the patient for the next two or three days against the same foodstuff.

Dr Joseph Miller runs the Miller Institute of Allergy in Mobil, Alabama, and is Clinical Associate Professor of Paediatrics at the University of Alabama College of Medicine in Birmingham, Alabama. Although Dr Miller readily accepts that he learnt the basic concept of this technique from Dr Carlton Lee, he applied his highly logical and ordered mind into extending and organizing this test so that it could be taught to other practitioners, nurses and technicians. He wrote the book *Provocative Testing and Injection Therapy* published by Charles C. Thomas (1972). This still remains the best teaching manual on this technique. As various physicians tried this technique they realized that the procedure could solve a wide range of problems that were hitherto insoluble. There are now a large number of clinics in the USA, a few in Australia and about eight clinics in the United Kingdom which are using this technique. A brief outline of this test follows.

Neutralization

Food extracts are obtained from the usual allergy supply companies in the standard one-in-ten or one-in-twenty prick-test concentrations containing glycerine. The dilutant that most clinics now use is benzyl alcohol, as it has a very low incidence of allergy in itself. The benzyl alcohol is prepared in intravenous-quality normal saline and, using this dilutant nine separate dilutions, a serial one-in-five dilution, are prepared. Thus dilutions of one in five, one in twenty-five, one in one hundred and twenty-five, one in six hundred and twenty-five, and so on are prepared for testing. The test consists of giving intradermal injections of varying concentrations of the foods known or suspected to be causing the patient's problems. Testing usually begins on one of the stronger strengths and, if a positive reaction is obtained, the doctor proceeds at ten-minute intervals to weaker strengths. Two things can happen during the course of these tests. On one hand, the original bleb produced by the intradermal injection, which we call a wheal, can increase in size indicating positivity. When positive wheals are obtained to foods, symptoms are often induced as well. These symptoms then normally become removed at the strength of food extract which produces a negative wheal.

In assessing wheals, there are various criteria. When 1/20 cc of a food extract is injected intradermally it will produce a wheal which, at the time of injection, is hard, raised, blanched and has well-demarcated edges. After ten minutes a positive wheal will usually have retained most of these features and will have grown at least 2 mm in diameter. Negative wheals lose these characteristics and grow less than 2 mm. If the initial injection results in a positive wheal, with or without symptoms, the physician moves to a consecutively weaker strength until the first negative wheal is found. This is the neutralizing dose and also the treatment concentration, unless symptoms induced by the stronger strength have not entirely cleared, in which case a move to the next weaker solution will normally clear them. In over 80 per cent of cases, the first negative wheal is the neutralizing dose. If a weaker dose than the neutralizing dose is administered, then symptoms will usually recur. This is called under-dosage and the symptoms can be removed by going back to the stronger dose which is obviously the neutralizing level. Thus, in a migraine patient, symptoms of headache which can be induced by too strong or too weak a dose can be removed by the neutralizing dose.

Patients find it amazing that their migraine and headache symptoms can be turned on and off within the space of a few minutes. Furthermore, this technique lends itself to fairly scientific valuation. The patient, of course, does not really know if the tester is using dummy (placebo) injections, for example normal saline. In our experience it is rare for a patient to react to such placebos and these reactions in general are almost always valid.

This account represents only the briefest outline of the technique and any reader who wishes to know more about it should read Dr Miller's book (see Further Reading). There are many concepts which are important for someone using this technique professionally to understand and these concepts include harmonic neutralizing doses, bound wheals, deutero wheals and so forth, which are not appropriate in this presentation.

After the neutralizing levels for the major food allergens have been determined, they are either administered to the patient by sublingual drops or by subcutaneous injections, which are usually self-administered. Sublingual drops are called this as they are placed beneath the tongue. The area under the human tongue has a good reputation for being an area of high absorbability. Inspection of the area under the tongue will reveal large veins which are called the sublingual veins and absorption into such blood vessels is effective in this area. This is, of course, the reason why patients who are taking nitrogylcerine tablets to treat angina place these tablets under their tongue to obtain the most rapid response. Sublingual desensitizing drops are hence placed under the tongue using a special dropper bottle and patients are taught how to do this correctly. The curved dropper bottles produce a carefully calibrated quantity and the solution in the dropper bottles is made up so that each single drop delivered from the pipette contains the precise neutralizing doses of the food to which the patient is sensitive. In other words, one drop delivered from such a bottle can contain neutralizing doses for a number of differing food allergens. Technicians use a fairly simple mathematical formula to calculate the amount of reagent each patient needs, dependent on the results of the skin testing. Sublingual drops are effective for about five hours, while subcutaneous injections will be effective for two days in most patients. The injections are normally made up in a 0.5 cc dosage and the amount of food allergens in these is of course calculated appropriately.

Of the two methods, my preference is for the subcutaneous injections although I do use both. Nowadays, modern insulin syringes are disposable, have a very fine inbuilt needle, are extremely easy to use and, most important of all, very rarely hurt the patient when he injects himself. Most patients who try both methods of administering their neutralizing doses prefer the injection because it is a little more effective, and the fact that it is only required every two days makes it very convenient. These desensitizing drops or injections fulfil two purposes. The first is that, within a day or so, they enable the patient to eat the food to which he is sensitive without adverse effect. Secondly, if the desensitization has been administered for a couple of years or so, the patient becomes desensitized to the food and finds he can eat it without recourse to his drops or injections.

This technique has already revolutionized the lives of many thousands of patients in the USA, Australia and in the United Kingdom. It is the only technique which allows the patient to eat the foods to which he is allergic without symptoms. It is in fact the most useful method that is currently in the hands of those allergists involved in the field of clinical ecology.

Diagnosis Using Skin-testing
An extension of this technique is to use it for diagnosis. Clearly, if positive wheal reactions and symptoms can be obtained in the course of desensitization, there is no need to put a patient through an elimination dietary procedure. Furthermore, whereas an elimination dietary procedure can take five or six weeks, during which time the patient in general has to avoid major social occasions, a comprehensive skin-testing programme can be completed in about four days of intensive testing. A workable procedure in these circumstances is to scan about 34 major foods in intradermal provocation skin tests. The patient's reaction to all 34 foods is tested and neutralizing doses are obtained for all those items to which there is a positive reaction. The testing procedure on average takes about seven 2½-hour test sessions to complete. At the end of the testing programme, the patient is allowed to eat only those foods tested and takes his injections or drops to cover all those items to which he has been found sensitive.

The advantages of this approach are considerable:

(1) The testing programme is completed in a few days.
(2) The patient does not have to assess his own response.
(3) The patient does not have to abandon his drugs and in some cases removing patients from their drugs can be either hazardous or extremely unpleasant.
(4) If the patient lives a long way from his clinic, this test

procedure saves him a whole series of long journeys at various stages of the elimination diet.

(5) If the patient has multiple food allergies, these tests will be inevitable anyway, even after the elmination diet, because the patient will need to be desensitized to a large number of foods.

(6) In most patients the treatment programme is very successful.

The disadvantages of this treatment, as opposed to the elimination diet followed by desensitization to specifically identified food allergens, are:

(1) The skin-test technique picks up adapted food allergies as well as non-adapted allergies (see Chapter 13). Hence the number of foods to which a patient reacts often appears more complicated than it really is. There is therefore a degree of over-treatment almost inevitably present using this technique.

(2) The patient does not know that he is going to become completely well until after the treatment is completed, whereas after the first stage of the elimination diet most patients can discover for themselves that, once removed from their major food allergies, they feel a completely different person.

(3) Going through an elimination diet probably gives the patient a better idea than skin testing as to which of his food allergens cause severe reactions and which mild, and also he may learn to associate certain symptoms with certain foods.

(4) The elimination diet is a decidedly educative programme, whereas skin testing is far less so in itself. Consequently, at the end of a skin-testing programme, the patient has to be educated into using only those items which have been tested. This involves some education into how multiple foods are made up and what they contain. For example, at the end of the testing programme, it is probable that wholemeal bread will be permitted in a patient's diet, but not white bread because the chemicals (bleaching agents, anti-staling agents, etc.) added to this have not been assessed. At the end of such a programme a patient can sabotage all the careful work that has been done up to that point by, for example, eating white bread. If he is sensitive to the chemicals in white bread and he is not covered for them by his desensitizing drops or

injections, this may in itself be enough to cause symptoms of migraine.

After remaining on the foods tested for a few weeks and presumably being free of migraines, the patient can then extend his repertoire of foods by bringing back into his diet one single food item at a time and testing it.

9

DESENSITIZATION AND OTHER TECHNIQUES FOR DEALING WITH INHALED ALLERGIES

In migraine the most common inhaled allergens are the various petrochemicals to which modern man is increasingly exposed. Reactions to the well-known non-chemical inhaled allergies such as house dust, house dust mite, various moulds, pollens and animal danders, can cause headache and migraine occasionally, but in my experience rarely. Certainly I have seen patients who have had headaches after the injection of specific mould extracts, which were then relieved by a neutralizing dose of the same mould. Such patients may well have headaches when the mould count becomes high. This may happen on humid days in August or September in the United Kingdom and especially just before a thunder storm. In these circumstances, the mould count soars dramatically and patients can notice headaches. The whole mould problem is usually inextricably connected with the intestinal thrush problem (see Chapter 7). The thrush in our intestines is stimulated by atmospheric moulds and is goaded into activity, producing whatever adverse symptoms the thrush produces in each individual patient.

Petrol and Diesel Fumes

By far the commonest inhalant producing headache or migraine is petrol and diesel fumes. Many hundreds of my patients will observe, 'If I drive up to central London to go shopping, I invariably get a headache or migraine.' Obviously the severity of the problem depends on factors like the intensity of the traffic and the heat of the day. The hotter the outside temperature, the more volatile the petrol and diesel fumes. Some patients are exquisitely sensitive to diesel exhaust fumes but far less so to petrol. These patients become very ill if stuck in a traffic jam immediately behind a bus or a lorry discharging large quantities of diesel exhaust directly into the ventilation systems of their cars. At my clinic we keep testing solutions for petrol exhaust fumes, diesel exhaust fumes and synthetic ethanol. Patients who have problems such as above are tested with these solutions, either intradermally (in the same way as we do for foods — see page 88-93) or sublingually. When we are testing intradermally, we look both for positive wheals associated with symptoms on the stronger levels, and then a negative wheal associated with the removal of symptoms when the neutralizing level is obtained. From the results of our intradermal testing we make up sublingual drops and patients can take these on such occasions as they are exposed to a high level of petrol or diesel fumes. The drops work usually for about two to four hours, depending on the level of pollution. Patients tend to keep their petrol/diesel desensitizing drops in their car so that they are always available if needed. The drops have a preventative effect on one hand and, in the event that the patient has forgotten to take the drops, they will help the patient to eradicate his/her symptoms, even after exposure. The petrol and diesel exhaust testing solutions are made by passing such fumes through glycerol saline and micropore filters. One disadvantage is that they are slightly unstable in solution and can deteriorate in time in terms of concentration. As concentration is critical, this can lead sometimes to diminished effectiveness.

Synthetic ethanol, which is ethyl alcohol made synthetically by condensation of ethylene gas, is much more stable in solution. Synthetic ethanol is, as Dr Randolph has said, a 'typical hydrocarbon' and is closely related to most of the main chemicals which cause problems with diesel and petrol exhaust fumes. Using synthetic ethanol as a testing solution and using the neutralizing doses so obtained is often more beneficial than using neutralizing doses of petrol or diesel exhaust, probably because of the stability of synthetic ethanol.

Negative Ionizers
While on the subject of car journeys, it is appropriate to mention that negative ionizers can often prove to be a helpful adjunct to the protection that many people need in their cars. Negative ionizers are made by many firms, often specifically for cars. They are designed to plug into the cigarette lighter

contact. As they use only 5 watts of power they take very little from the battery and most patients leave them plugged in all the time that their ignition is on. Beneficial response to these devices varies quite a lot and as a result of this most firms that manufacture them will return the cost of these devices to their customers if they prove unsatisfactory.

That negative ionizers are effective in reducing pollution was recently demonstrated in the United States of America. A room was filled with a certain concentration of cigarette smoke and the smoke allowed gradually to clear itself. This took about 36 hours. The same room was later filled with the same amount of smoke and a negative ionizer used. In these circumstances the concentration of smoke fell to the same level in about 50 minutes.

A minor snag with the use of negative ionizers is the observation that walls of rooms become much more discoloured than usual. The negative ionizer causes pollutants normally attached to positive ions to go to the nearest positive source, i.e. the walls of the room. Although this causes minor problems with decorating, it does at least demonstrate that the device is effective.

Air depollution units are used by many people within their homes to considerable effect. As far as I know, there have been none developed for use in cars. The ventilation systems of cars vary considerably. A few models draw in very little air from the outside, and this may be helpful for some individuals.

Some patients, interestingly, seem to gain a fair degree of protection from the inhalent problem by the use of sodium cromoglycate. This medication is most commonly known as Intal and has been extensively used by asthmatics for many years. Sodium cromoglycate is quite different from most medications in that it is a true preventative drug and not just a symptom modifier. It works by 'coating' the mast cells in the lining of the lungs and the nasal passages, which initiate the allergic response. In other words, it works by stopping the allergens really getting at the patient. For the most satisfactory effect, we find a combination of Lomusol and Intal is needed. Lomusol is the nasal form of the medication and is instilled into the nose by drops. Intal protects the mast cells in the lining of the lung and is administered by an inhaler.

Most patients find a combination of one or more of the above suggestions to be very helpful.

Common Inhalants

Other common intermittently inhaled problems are cigarette smoke, formaldehyde, perfumes, paint fumes, phenol (soft plastics), varnishes and tar.

The cigarette smoke problem is best helped by avoidance and of course over the past few years more and more forms of public transportation and places of entertainment have recognized that people have a right not to inhale other people's cigarette smoke and have made some attempt to separate smokers and non-smokers. When such avoidance is not possible, desensitization, sodium cromoglycate, negative ionizers and all the other suggestions can prove helpful.

Formaldehyde is an extremely commonly encountered problem. For most people the contact that is most obvious is fabric shops where there is a peculiarly high concentration of formaldehyde used in the manufacture of these fabrics. Other common contacts with formaldehyde are air fresheners, home heating insulation, chipboard, permanent-press clothes, toothpaste and shampoos. Although headache is a symptom tht can emanate from formaldehyde, perhaps more commonly it irritates the eyes, the nose and the throat. It has been calculated that about one fifth of the entire population is affected to some extent by the presence of this chemical (reported in *The Washington Post*, 25 March, 1980). A few patients may have enormous problems with constant exposure to ureaformaldehyde foam used as a cavity wall insulation. Once installed, this is extremely difficult to get rid of. Exposure to such constant sources of problem does not result, as far as I am aware, in specific migraines, but it can lead to a constant background headiness and muzziness.

Perfumes are a major source of headaches to many people. Often specific types will upset various individuals, but some are upset by all perfumes. Avoidance or specific desensitization are again the more useful techniques available to help these patients.

Paint fumes are in general not too much of a problem for most patients. Certain paints, especially gloss paint which contains toluene, can give susceptible individuals a splitting headache. However, within a few days most paints out-gas to a level at which they do not affect most individuals. Exquisitely sensitive patients may react for very much longer. One helpful suggestion for many people is to use paints with a silk finish rather than a gloss as there is no toluene in silk-finish paints.

Plastics, especially soft plastics, give off a gas called phenol. Phenol is also the main constituent of disinfectants such as are used in hospitals and dental surgeries. Departmental stores with large amounts of soft plastics will, particularly if the temperature is high, give quite a lot of patients muzzy headaches or other similar symptoms. Again desensitization or sodium cromoglycate can be helpful in these circumstances.

Domestic Gas and Oil

Domestic gas and oil, especially gas, are the commonest problems encountered by patients suffering from chemical sensitivity. The exposure to these chemicals is virtually continuous in patients who have appliances such as gas central heating boilers, oil boilers or gas cookers in their house. As these hydrocarbons are burnt within the confines of the home, the levels which are attained are not diluted by large quantities of air and remain in measurable quantities several days after all such appliances are turned off at the mains. Even if the appliances are only situated in the kitchen, the pollution extends right throughout the house in surprisingly high levels.

Outdoor air pollution has always excited more interest in both professional and lay minds, but indoor air pollution is in fact vastly more important because of the level of pollution attained and the constancy of exposure. Constant levels of gas or oil probably rarely cause specific attacks of migraine, but can induce a wide range of symptoms of a chronic nature. I have seen a large number of cases of rheumatoid arthritis where gas has been a major factor and many other polysymptomatic conditions. There are many cases when gas has been implicated in a constant or near constant background headiness or muzziness. Furthermore, because of the 'barrel effect', patients who have these sensitivities to gas and oil never feel particularly well, even if their food sensitivity problems are elucidated. If exposure to such a constant problem continues, despite it being only one out of many, all sorts of other problems tend to occur.

The most common one is that neutralizing levels to foods can change, sometimes with great frequency. The other problem is that in these circumstances, new food sensitivities can develop with alarming frequency. Some allergists have a theory that there is a 'gate-keeper' allergy which, once it occurs, tends to open the flood-gates to other allergies. If this is a valid concept, then certainly gas is frequently a gate-keeper allergy. Perhaps more likely, though, gas may have a general toxic effect on the enzyme systems of susceptible people, leading to the development of additional food sensitivities.

Identification of this problem is usually accomplished in various stages. A history of adverse reactions to various intermittently-inhaled hydrocarbons, such as petrol, paint and perfumes, should alert the physician to the possibility of adverse reactions to gas. It is rare in my experience for patients to have noticed before they see us that gas affects them, and this is presumably due to the constancy of exposure. Once suspicion has been aroused, the next stage consists of intradermal testing using reagents such as synthetic ethanol and gas exhaust. The development of a positive wheal reaction to these reagents, particularly if accompanied by symptoms on the high dosage levels, is excellent evidence of a positive problem with gas. The symptoms should, of course, be subsequently 'turned off' when the neutralizing level is reached and may again become worse when a dose weaker than the neutralizing level is tried. When this sequence of events occurs, there is really no doubt, but such obvious reactions are not always seen, even in cases which are subsequently proven to be genuine.

The ultimate test is to turn off all gas or oil utilities for about seven to ten days, with extensive ventilation of the house to eliminate existing gas or oil residues. If constant symptoms are removed in such circumstances and then recur on re-establishing the gas or oil supply, the evidence is quite complete. If there is any doubt, of course, the whole procedure can be repeated, if necessary two or three times. As some houses lose a little gas from their pipes and around the gas meter, an even better test is for the patient to spend a week in an all-electric house. Apart from other considerations, as gas has never been present in such a house, symptoms clear more quickly. It is obvious that in the house where gas has been present, there will be some continuation of symptoms while the remnants of the gas are being ventilated away.

In any patient in whom gas or oil sensitivity is confirmed, there is only one satisfactory course of action and this is the complete eradication of gas or oil burning from the interior of the house. This means the replacement of gas cookers and fires by electric ones. However, the most expensive item is the re-siting of the gas or oil boiler. Most gas/oil boilers are situated in kitchens or airing cupboards. If a patient is gas/oil-sensitive, such boilers must be situated outside the house and this is a procedure which inevitably costs several hundreds of pounds, depending on whether there is already an outhouse separated from the house by at least one foot of clean air.

There are several situations when such a move is impossible, for example if the patient lives in a fourth-floor flat and has no garden. Other examples include listed buildings in which outhouses are not allowed for planning reasons. In such circumstances, the patient has the stark choice of an inevitable continuation of his illness or a change of address.

To summarize, therefore, it is not impossible to deal with the chemical problem in the atmosphere. Most of the problems turn out to be indoor air pollution and the removal of gas, soft plastics and other such items can solve this aspect. Outdoor air pollution can be dealt with using desensitization and other techniques.

10.
EVIDENCE THAT NEUTRALIZATION WORKS

In this chapter I will attempt to outline the evidence that these approaches to testing and neutralizing allergies are valid. To those physicians who are in daily contact with patients undergoing treatment it is obvious that it is effective, as almost all patients report that since receiving their desensitizing injections, they are able to eat foods which previously upset them. Alternatively, they report that they are able to cope with inhalants that previously upset them. There have been various clinical trials, all of them carried out in the United States of America, which have supported this view. It must first be emphasized that in these trials the food allergies that were being neutralized and desensitized were not limited to ones causing migraine, although a proportion of the patients being assessed in this way were migraine sufferers. I think, however, it is reasonable to assume, that, if the effects of a food can be neutralized, it probably does not matter whether that food is causing migraine, fatigue, eczema, asthma, colitis or whatever.

Intradermal Testing and Neutralization
The first clinical trial to demonstrate the validity of neutralization therapy was organized by Dr Joseph Miller of Mobile, Alabama. The trial was published in the *Annals of Allergy*, Volume No. 38, No. 3, March 1977 and entitled, 'A Double-blind Study of Food Extract Injection Therapy'. Dr Miller was, as described earlier, the physician most connected with clarifying, organizing and teaching this concept in the first place.

Patients who were selected for this study had illnesses strongly suspected to be due to food sensitivity. Each patient was extensively tested for all their commonly-eaten foods by intradermal provocation neutralization testing. The neutralizing doses of the implicated foods were combined into a single injection solution specifically for each individual patient. The injections were self-administered subcutaneously daily for twenty days. Patients were restricted to eating those foods that had been assessed.

Placebo injections were prepared which were indistinguishable in appearance, etc. from the injections containing the active neutralizing doses. The placebo injections were also self-administered daily for twenty days. The first series of injections to be used (active or placebo) was decided randomly by the toss of a coin by a third party. Thus, neither the patient nor the physician were aware of which extracts were employed. This trial, therefore, qualifies for the title of a double-blind trial. In the summary it was stated that the superiority of active extract over placebo extract for the eight patients involved was clearly significant at a 99.8% level of confidence. In most patients the active extract was rapidly and markedly effective and the placebo was totally ineffective.

Case No. 1, for example, was a 29-year-old white female with severe migraine problems recurrent since early childhood, becoming progressively worse. In the preceding six months the headaches had wakened her in the early morning hours every day. She reported that headaches followed the ingestion of coffee, chocolate, beef, pork and ice-cream amongst other things. She had been taking potent drugs by mouth and potent injections for nine years. Additional symptoms included recurrent vertigo, buzzing in the ears, nausea, abdominal cramps and depression.

The first series of injections administered was of active extract. After the third injection she required no further medication and was completely free of headache, vertigo, tinnitus and depression for the remainder of the twenty days. She stated that this was the longest period she had ever gone without a headache in her entire life. The nausea and abdominal cramps were present very mildly. On the second series of injections (placebo) the headaches and all her other symptoms returned on the fourth day and remained severe for the rest of the twenty days. On the third series of injections (active) her symptoms had almost cleared by the third day and she remained virtually symptom-free for the rest of the twenty-day period. On the fourth series (placebo) her symptoms returned again but not as severely as on the second series. This is a common finding in this type of trial. By the time the second placebo phase has started the patient has had forty desensitizing injections during the two active phases and the patient is beginning to become desensitized. This desensitizing effect carries over into the placebo phase, despite discontinuation of the active injections and provides some carry-over protection. Although this is evidence that a long-term desensitization effect occurs, it tends to diminish the difference between the active and placebo phases and thus understates the advantage of the active extract.

Case No. 3 in this study was also a severe migraine sufferer aged 57. She had had severe migraine accompanied by nausea and vomiting since early childhood which had become progressively worse in the seven months prior to the study. She had been awakened by severe headaches every morning at 4 a.m. She had very frequent injections of narcotics such as pethidine in high dosage. Every three weeks or so these injections failed her and she was hospitalized and heavily sedated for three to seven days. She herself did not think it was likely that foods were related to her migraine. The first series of injections (placebo) did not beneficially affect her at all. In the second series (active) the headaches became noticeably less severe after the third injection. Her photophobia and acne also became markedly better. Only a few mild headaches and one migraine occurred in the twenty-days' evaluation period. On the third series (placebo) she went rapidly downhill and by the sixth day her pethidine was no longer able to control her symptoms and she was re-admitted to hospital for five days. The headaches continued in their original severity and frequency for the balance of the twenty days. On the fourth series (active) she noticed improvement again on the fifth day and had no severe headaches for the rest of this phase.

Case No. 5 in this series was another migraine sufferer, this one aged 52, and she had suffered from migraine for the preceding twenty-five years. The migraines were severe and lasted two to three days at a time. In addition she suffered from nausea, vertigo, faints, laryngeal oedema, flatulence, diarrhoea, eczema and urticaria. On the first series (active) her headaches and all other symptoms cleared after the third injection and remained clear throughout this phase. In the second (placebo) phase most symptoms returned by Day 7. On the third series (active) the headaches and flatulence cleared after the first injection and all symptoms remained clear for the rest of this phase. On the fourth series (placebo) all symptoms continued to remain clear, again demonstrating the long-term desentizing effect noted earlier.

I have selected these three cases from the eight studied, largely because they were severe migraine sufferers, but also because they were typical of the benefit demonstrated in all eight cases.

In April 1984 Dr William J. Rea and his colleagues at the Environmental Health Centre in Dallas reported a similar trial in the *Archives of Otolaryngology*, which was entitled 'Elimination of Oral Food Challenge Reactions by Ingestion of Food Extracts.' This trial was in my opinion attempting to do something rather more difficult than that which had been demonstrated in Dr Miller's trial. Dr Rea was attempting to turn off deliberately-induced food-allergic reactions with a single neutralizing dose of that food. As demonstrated in Dr Miller's trial several sequential daily injections were often required before maximum benefit was obtained. I know this also from my own experience.

In their comment on the trial the authors wrote in summary that the results of this study were consistent with previous double-blind studies in providing support for the existence of the neutralizing dose effect that is different from and superior to the effect of the placebo. The responses in terms of signs and symptoms were divided into six different possible variables. For each of these six variables a very significant difference was found between the neutralization and placebo situations. This demonstrated the effectiveness of the neutralizing dose in relief of symptomatology. The return of oral food challenge reactions when the placebo injections were used further emphasized the validity of the neutralizing dose method. Extremely elaborate precautions were taken to make these tests absolutely foolproof in terms of the double-blind, etc. and full details of this are given in the original paper. The paper concluded with the statement that, 'It appears that the phenomenon of subcutaneous food neutralization can be scientifically endorsed for clinical use in the treatment of food reactions.'

Another study of neutralizing therapy was published in the *Journal of Learning Disabilities* in April 1984. The authors were Dr James O'Shea and Dr S. F. Porter. The purpose of the study was to determine by double-blind study whether the hyperkinetic syndrome (better known in England as hyperactivity) in children was at least partly due to individual reactions to foods, dyes and inhalants. After being assessed by intradermal and sublingual testing, composite individual extracts were provided for each patient. As in Dr Miller's trial an active phase and a placebo phase was employed. Each child's behaviour in each phase was monitored by parents, teachers and a psychologist. Significant improvement was noticed in eleven out of the fourteen children when treated with the active preparations as opposed to the placebos.

In the field of inhaled allergy problems there has, as yet, been only one published trial relating to neutralization therapy. This trial was published in the *Journal of Allergy and Clinical Immunology* in 1983. The authors were Drs Boris Schiff, Weindorf and Inselman. This particular trial was carried out entirely in the laboratory. In the summary the authors stated that the effect of neutralizing therapy on patients who had asthma induced by reactions to animal fur were evaluated using peak flow meters and other similar instruments. All patients were first of all challenged with increasing amounts of animal fur dander until the amount required to cause a 20 per cent decrease in the peak flow was determined. Neutralizing levels were then obtained in the traditional way to the specific animal fur danders that were being used. The patients were given either no treatment, placebo treatment or active neutralization treatment. The results showed that the FEV 1 (forced expiratory volume in one second) decreased 27.7 per cent from baseline in the controls, 25.9 per cent after placebo injections, but only 9.4 per cent after the active neutralizing injections. They concluded that there was a distinct diminution in animal dander-induced bronchospasm with neutralization therapy, which may well have important therapeutic implications. These results are particularly good when it is considered that this improvement resulted from one single injection. As the previously-quoted trials have demonstrated, there is a build-up effect after several injections have been given.

Sublingual Provocation Trials

There have been several other reports relating to the efficacy and validity of sublingual testing for food allergies. These trials have not concerned themselves with the neutralization aspect, but have concentrated on whether patients can distinguish between a placebo and a sublingually-administered extract of a food to which they are sensitive. As indicated earlier, my view is that sublingual testing is markedly inferior to intradermal testing as it relies entirely on the patient's subjective response, both for diagnosis and also for determination of the neutralizing level. The intradermal test has also the wheal appearance, indicating positivity or negativity, which is extremely helpful because, of course, it is independent of the patient's subjective feelings. Furthermore, I have the impression clinically that some foods are not absorbed well under the tongue and that this is a potent cause of inaccuracy. In 1981 the *Journal of Biological Psychiatry* published a paper by Dr D. King entitled 'Can Allergic Exposure Provoke Psychological Symptoms? A Double-blind Test.' This trial evaluated allergy patients who had at least one psychological symptom, such as anxiety, depression, confusion or problem with concentration. The question to be determined was, 'Did sublingual provocation with a specific food induce psychological symptoms more frequently than a placebo?' Thirty patients were challenged with selected foods and with triple-distilled water as a placebo. The trial was subdivided into four types of trial: (1) Allergen trials — four allergy-producing foods each given three times. (2) Placebo trials — two tests each given three times. (3) Base rate trials in which the subjects received nothing sublingually but nevertheless received a complete evaluation. (4) Open placebo trials to assess any biological reactivity of the placebo (three trials). Great care was taken to ensure that the test was properly double-blind, including the evaluation. Average symptom scores for psychological symptoms were four times higher after allergy-producing foods than after placebo provocation. The difference was highly statistically significant ($P = 0.001$). Therefore Dr King would appear to have demonstrated that challenge sublingually with foods known to produce allergy can produce psychological symptoms much more frequently than placebo.

In July 1982 Dr Marshall Mandell and Dr A. Conte had a paper published in the *Journal of the International Academy of*

Preventive Medicine. It was called, 'The Role of Allergy in Arthritis, Rheumatism and Polysymptomatic Cerebral, Visceral and Somatic Disorders. A Double-blind Study.' The paper described the reactions of thirty patients with arthritic pain. Each patient received a sublingual challenge of nineteen food allergy-producing items, five inhalants and four placebos of distilled water. The positive symptomatic response rate was 61 per cent for foods, 38 per cent for the inhalants and 6.6 per cent for the placebos. Each of these differences was highly significant statistically.

It must be noted in all fairness at this point that there have been two trials of provocative sublingual testing which have shown totally negative results. However, both trials were carried out in such a way that a positive outcome was virtually impossible.

In 1980 the *Annals of Allergy* published a study by Dr C. Lehman. He attempted to demonstrate whether sublingual food challenges would induce changes in the oedema and swelling of the mucous membrane of the nose and compared this with the response to placebo drops. This study showed a totally negative correlation, but the choice of one single parameter to measure (i.e. the nasal mucous membrane) was a fundamental mistake. In most clinical circumstances the assessment of clinical response will include several clinical variables. As Dr Lehman himself admitted, 'The nasal mucosal oedema is constantly changing at ten-minute intervals to other appearances quite independent of whether foods or anything else are placed under the tongue.' Thus the choice of such a fluctuant and unstable measure invalidates any conclusion, positive or negative, that this trial could produce. However, more important, and in my view amazingly, the patients were not even known to be allergic to the specific foods that were tested. The patients apparently only had some 'history of food allergy'. Prior specific sensitivity was only suspected for eleven out of the sixty foods that were challenged. This makes the trial a complete nonsense, as for most of the time patients' reactions to a food to which they were not even allergic were being compared with a placebo.

The same sort of criticism applies to the 1973 report of the Food Allergy Committee of the American Academy of Allergy. Their subjects were supposed to have a 'known allergy to at least one of the five foods to be surveyed', but the actual number that were sensitive to each specific food was never reported. If, for example, each subject was actually sensitive to only one of the five test foods, a 20 per cent average response rate for food allergens would be expected. As there was a high placebo response rate in any case in this study, one would hardly expect a 20 per cent response rate to show any advantage over a placebo. There were in addition several other major omissions and methodological errors which completely, in my view, invalidated this report. Incredibly, only three out of the ten participating physicians had any experience whatsoever with sublingual provocation testing. It must be said that one is forced to wonder about the motivation of those involved in this trial.

Setting up clinical trials is a complex subject and needs to be done with great precision. Testing for food allergy needs a certain expertise, as do most medical tests. Those trials which have been reported by physicians who have been careful to take the precaution of identifying specific food allergies and other similar extremely critical factors precisely, have all shown positive results for the identification of food sensitivities by sublingual testing. Thus, the results of the trials that have been done well have shown very positive proof that sublingual testing is valuable.

In regard to the main factor, that is whether intradermal testing and neutralization is effective, there have been no published trials which one can set against the very positive results detailed earlier in this chapter. Although it would be nice to have yet further proof of the validity of neutralization and intradermal testing, as things stand at the moment the evidence we have for it is extremely good.

11.

OTHER METHODS OF DIAGNOSING AND TREATING FOOD ALLERGIES

Testing Food Allergies
We shall now survey methods used by some physicians for testing for food allergy which have not been discussed elsewhere in this book.

These are:

(a) prick skin testing
(b) the R.A.S.T. test (radio allergo sorbent test)
(c) cytotoxic test
(d) kinesiology
(e) radionics
(f) sublingual food testing

Tests (a) and (b) are still frequently used by conventional allergists, but they both suffer from serious defects. Tests (c), (d) and (e) are frowned on by most conventionally-trained allergists and by most clinical ecologists. Test (f) is used by some clinical ecologists, but is generally regarded as similar but inferior to the intradermal provocation skin test.

(a) Prick testing
This is a fairly useful test for inhalant allergies but does not really help in the diagnosis of food allergy. It is this simple fact which has, in my opinion, held back until recently the development of interest in food allergy.

The test involves placing a single drop of allergen extract on the inner forearm. A lancet is introduced through the drop of extract on the skin at an acute angle and, having slightly penetrated the skin, is given a deliberate vertical lift before being removed. Responses to these tests are read after ten to twenty minutes. Many of these tests can be performed within a few minutes of each other and this test therefore is both simple and quick to perform. Unhappily, as I have already said, it is not very effective and most patients with well-established food allergies will fail to react posititively to this test. As clinical ecologists have become familiar with the intradermal provocative neutralizing test, it has become apparent why prick tests are so useful for diagnosing inhalant allergies but not for food allergies. Comparison between prick tests and varying strengths of intradermal wheals shows that the No. 4 strength intradermal is approximately equivalent to a positive prick test. In other words, if a patient is positive on the No. 1, 2 and 3 strength of the intradermal provocation test but negative on the 4 level, he will have a negative prick test to that same item. In practice, the neutralizing point (the strongest negative wheal) for most inhalants is around the 5, 6 or 7 level, so they could be expected to have positive prick tests. In the case of foods, however, the common neutralizing points are the 2, 3 and 4 levels. These would all therefore be negative on prick test. Only patients who neutralize on the 5 level or weaker could be anticipated to react positively to prick tests. Prick tests are therefore not only ineffective but are at times positively harmful. I have known of patients with genuine food allergies who have been informed categorically that their allergies do not exist, purely on the basis of this test.

(b) The RAST test (radio allergo sorbent test)

This particular test involves taking a blood sample and measuring the quantity of immunoglobulin E antibodies that form when this blood is exposed to different allergens. It is thought that the higher the count of IgE antibodies, the more allergic the patient. The RAST test is fairly useful in diagnosing allergies to dust, dust mite, moulds, animal danders, pollens and some foods. It has, however, many drawbacks: (1) It can only be used for testing a very limited number of food allergies. (2) It costs about five times more per allergy tested than does provocative neutralization testing. (3) It measures only immediate responses and many food-allergic reactions are delayed. (4) RAST tests take a few days before results are available. Provocative neutralization skin testing results are available almost immediately. (5) Interpretation and technique vary somewhat from laboratory to laboratory and false negatives and false positives often occur. (6) It is quite probable that in the future the RAST test may be refined and become more useful. However, at its best, even if this does happen, the only therapeutic approach that will stem from it would be dietary avoidance of the incriminated foods with all its attendant difficulties and disadvantages. Comparative tests done in the United States between RAST and provocative intradermal neutralization have shown that the provocative neutralization testing is superior and of course it has the inestimable advantage of enabling the patient to eat the foods to which he is sensitive.

(c) Cytotoxic Testing
This is just about the most controversial of all tests for food allergy. There are a few physicians who enthusiastically promote this test, but the whole of the conventional allergy establishment and most clinical ecologists are very sceptical about its value. It does, of course, have the superficial attraction of suggesting that countless food and chemical allergies can be diagnosed from a single sample of intravenous blood. The term cytotoxic literally means 'having a toxic effect on cells.' The blood sample is incubated on a microscope slide with a weak solution of suspected food allergen and the effect on certain specific white cells is noted. In a positive test the polymorph leucocytes (one type of white cell) slow down, become rounded and, in strongly positive cases, disintegrate. There is no doubt that this phenomenon occurs, but the interpretation of these results depends on the varying judgment of different technicians. One criticism of this method is that results may vary very substantially in the same patient from week to week or even from day to day. Perhaps with greater refinement and standardization, results may become more reliable. In the meantime, it cannot be denied that some patients have become well when they have adopted the diet suggested by these tests.

The E.N.T. Hospital of Helsinki University has used this test since 1975 and the doctors there report that it gives useful clues as to where to start their investigations. Dr Damien Downing, who has researched this technique very thoroughly, claims a 70 per cent reliability for the method but I am not sure how he obtains this figure and what he considers 100 per cent reliability to be. Having seen a number of patients over the years who have had this test, I have had the impression that I could obtain roughly the same results by what I might call the 'good guess method'. This method involves taking a history, which includes a diet history, from the patient. From this one can establish which foods the patient eats most often and, combining this information with the knowledge that certain foods are frequent offenders in certain conditions, one might well correctly guess which foods are the particular problem. This method, however, will frequently fail and, rather than mess around with measures such as this, I prefer to use techniques which have a very high success rate, even though the patient may have more of a problem with his diet initially. The biggest criticism of the cytotoxic test, and in my opinion a fair one, is that companies offering the test often do so directly to the patient. Sometimes they appear to discover huge numbers of food sensitivities and as a result some patients might end up on a very harsh and possibly nutritionally-inadequate diet, totally unsupervised by anyone with any knowledge of nutrition. Of course, this situation arises partly because most physicians in the NHS stubbornly refuse to have any involvement with this field at all.

(d) Applied kinesiology
This method is particularly favoured by chiropractors, some of whom have taken an interest in the field of food allergy. Initially, the practitioner establishes the patient's muscle strength and tone by observing how easily he can lift, for example, a 50lb weight. An allergen is introduced, usually under the tongue, and the muscle tone again measured. The theory is that an allergic reaction will weaken the muscle tone and this can be detected by the practitioner. There may be something in this test, but there has been absolutely no scientific validation of it as yet. At the moment, as there are relatively well-validated alternatives in existence, I feel that these approaches should be used in preference to applied kinesiology.

(e) Radionics
Several people in the United Kingdom claim to be able to diagnose food allergies from hair samples. A pendulum is dangled over the hair sample and, if it rotates in one way allergy is indicated, and if it is in the opposite way it is not. Although I accept that there are several very strange magnetic phenomena which we do not yet understand, this particular

test stretches credibility to breaking point. I have had many patients who have seen me after they have been tested in this way and the allergies that we have detected have borne little relationship to their hair test results.

The worst aspect of fringe tests such as cytotoxic testing, kinesiology and radionics, is that many physicians who are dubious about the concept of food sensitivity have seized upon these tests and their complete lack of scientific validation to criticize serious allergists and clinical ecologists who, in fact, do not use these tests anyway.

(f) Sublingual testing
When I was first interested in the subject of food allergy, I did quite a lot of tests using this method. The principle is the same as the intradermal provocative test. Solutions are made up in nine separate concentrations with a 1 in 5 dilution factor between one strength and another. The first strength is the strongest, the second is one-fifth weaker and so on and so forth. The technique consists of placing one measured drop of the food to be tested under the patient's tongue using a specially-designed dropper pipette. The area under the tongue is one of great absorbability as the large sublingual veins are present there. The patient lies quietly on a couch and any resulting symptoms are noted. It is also usual to take the pulse and record the size of the pupils at intervals. If symptoms or other changes occur, successively weaker levels are administered until they are counteracted. A more elaborate description of this technique can be found in Richard Mackarness' book *Not All in the Mind* (Pan Books).

Sometimes, particularly with very soluble foodstuffs such as milk, tea, coffee, orange, etc., one can see dramatic and obvious reactions when these are introduced under the tongue. With less soluble items, particularly items such as wheat and corn, reactions can easily fail to materialize despite the fact that the patient has a wheat or corn sensitivity and I cannot recall seeing anyone in their middle ages who has had a dramatic reaction to wheat, corn or any other cereal given sublingually.

The other disadvantage is that it is much more difficult to obtain the neutralizing level when foods are tested in this way. This form of testing is inferior to intradermal provocation testing, as intradermal provocation testing has two pillars on which the assessment can be made. One pillar represents the symptoms which are being induced or relieved. The other pillar is the appearance of the wheal. These two facets complement each other and the wheal changes normally correlate with the changes in symptom pattern. With some patients, however, with allergies identified as a result of the elimination diet, the sublingual testing, or even the intradermal testing, will fail to induce any symptoms whatsoever. With the intradermal testing one at least can observe the wheat response, but with sublingual testing one just has to record the test as negative although earlier testing has proved that there was a positive reaction.

Treatments for Food Allergies

The two fairly well-established forms of treatment for food allergies are: provocative intradermal neutralization treatment given either by injection or by sublingual drops and validated by trials mentioned in Chapte 8, or the anti-Candida treatment mentioned in Chapter 7. This does not have the same degree of validation as neutralization therapy, but experience of physicans using this treatment has been so spectacular in some patients that we regard this treatment as well proven. Other forms of treatment which have been employed at times are: (1) auto-immune urine therapy; (2) acupuncture and acu-pressure; (3) homoeopathy.

(1) Auto-immune urine therapy

This therapy was originally introduced in 1947 and has a small number of enthusiastic advocates. The technique consists of collecting the patient's urine the morning after he has eaten a meal containing all the items to which he suspects or knows that he is sensitive. The urine is filtered through micropore filters and is injected in specific and increasing quantities into the patient, usually into his thigh. A variation on this technique is to titrate the patient to his own urine' intradermally and to find a neutralizing level in the same way as is done with foods. The neutralizing dose can then either be taken by injection or sublingual drops.

This treatment has a valid immunological basis as many antigens are excreted in the urine. By subsequently reintroducing them back into the body it is possible to build up the level of T-lymphocytes, which is the best single indicator of the competence of the patient's immunologic system. However, antigens from the kidneys are also being re-injected and this can cause the immune system to start repelling its own tissue. As this can be very damaging to the kidneys, auto-immune urine injection therapy is a procedure to be avoided.

(2) Acupuncture and acupressure

This ancient Chinese healing art claims to be able to heal an enormous variety of mental and physical ailments. The theory is that the body's energy passes along imaginary lines called meridians. These meridians supposedly connect sensitive areas under the skin with diseased internal organs which are often situated a long way away from these specific skin sites. These meridian lines are not explainable by any Western knowledge of anatomy or physiology. The treatment entails inserting long thin needles into these specific sensitive areas. The needles remain in situ for about twenty or thirty minutes and there is some variation in the way in which the needles are used. Sometimes they are twirled, sometimes wired to electrical currents and sometimes pre-heated.

Recent work completed in Scotland has shown that stimulating certain points on the body also stimulates the pituitary gland in the brain. This in turn can produce chemicals called endorphins. These chemicals resemble various narcotics in their effect and can relieve pain and produce a general sense of well-being. It may well be this effect which accounts for the benefit that many patients find with acupuncture.

(3) Migraine and homoeopathy

Homoeopathy is a system of medicine developed by Dr Samuel Hahnemann at the end of the eighteenth century. Homoeopathy makes use of minute quantities of naturally-occurring substances, which, if taken in a larger dose, might actually precipitate symptoms similar, if not identical, to those one is trying to treat.

A particularly good example in relation to migraine, is coffee. When taken to excess, this can precipitate a headache, which may also occur on its withdrawal. Some coffee users will find that taking one or two cups of coffee may actually improve their migraine! This is certainly true if it is a 'withdrawal' headache. Whilst coffee is not recommended as a treatment for migraine, it is true to say that many people with migraine derive benefit from homoeopathic remedies. Below are four commonly used remedies for migraine, and the type of headaches which they may benefit most:

Nux vomica: For pain over the eyes, with sensitivity to light and sound. The person is often irritable and the headache may have been precipitated by excess food or drink.

Bryonia: For a bursting, splitting headache, particularly at the back of the head, associated with thirst and dryness of the mouth.

Aconite: For a heavy, bursting headache, associated with fear and anxiety. Migraine precipitated by shock, or of sudden onset, may be an indication for the use of Aconite.

Phosphoric acid: This may help a headache that is crushing, or characterized by pressure on the top of the head, particularly if the patient is tired or exhausted by the headache.

There are many other remedies that can be prescribed by doctors and practitioners conversant with homoeopathy.

Homoeopathy should never be considered as a substitute for finding the cause of one's migraine. Homoeopathic remedies can be used very easily by the patient, without fear of side-effects, and if the patient is on an exclusion diet, they will not upset the interpretation of the patient's response to the exclusion diet, in the way that taking an aspirin might. However, in some cases they might have, for example, lactose as a filler or binding agent, and this might confuse an elimination diet. The liquid forms are generally free of such problems.

Further information on homoeopathic prescribing can be obtained from the Homoeopathic Development Foundation, Harcourt House, 19a Cavendish Square, London W1M 9AD, telephone 01-629 3205. Details of doctors practising homoeopathy can be obtained from the Faculty of Homoeopathy, Royal London Homoeopathic Hospital, Great Ormond Street, London WC1N 3HR, telephone 01-837 3091.

In this chapter I have described several approaches which differ from the conventional medical point of view. I have given my current view of these techniques, but I am well aware of the fact that I may well modify these views as time goes on and more work is done with them. All these methods of testing and treatment have enthusiastic advocates. It is likely that there is some benefit to be derived from any of them, and the fact that we cannot fully comprehend or explain these phenomena does not mean that they are invalid.

All Science Starts with Observation

If a rational explanation cannot be obtained for an observation is does not necessarily mean that the observation is wrong. There is a terrible tendency in Western medicine, however, to take this attitude and nothing could be more calculated to stop progress. If a rational explanation cannot be found at first, more efforts should be made until one is found. Then, in turn, this may very well reveal further truths.

I would like to thank Dr Alan Stewart of Hove, Sussex, for help with the section on homoeopathy.

12.

THE MIGRAINE TRIALS

This book opened with a brief summary of a recent trial that has been published investigating the interrelationship of food allergy and migraine. This particular trial, by Professor Soothill and his colleagues, is in my view the best yet published and to my mind conclusively proves the case. Over the years, however, there has been a large number of trials. The early ones all originated from the United States of America but the last five trials have come from separate London teaching hospitals. There now follows a brief outline of the earlier trials, followed by a more detailed analysis of the five British trials to discover just what they tell us. It will be noted that, apart from a brief mention of the hydrocarbon problem in Dr Grant's trial and in that of the Hospital for Sick Children at Great Ormond Street this aspect of allergy has only been superficially studied and it is probable that some of the failures mentioned in these trials resulted from chemical susceptibility. The main problem in conducting trials is that editors of medical journals like their authors to concentrate their fire on one aspect, for example food allergy, and report whatever contribution this single factor has in the production of migraine. This is all right as far as it goes, but it tends to distract attention away from other important factors such as chemical susceptibility and the intestinal candida problem.

The first physician to report on the correlation of food and migraine was Dr Liveing in 1873, who wrote a classic account of migraine entitled 'On Megrim, Sick Headaches and Some Allied Disorders'. He reported that certain articles of diet occasionally act as 'exciting causes of the seizures'. He mentioned wine and burnt pastry as causes of some migraine.

A number of other physicians, such as Dr W. T. Vaughan,

reported many individual cases of food allergy in migraine sufferers, but Dr Albert Rowe of southern California was the first to complete a fairly extensive organized migraine trial. In 1928 in the *Journal of California and Western Medicine,* he recorded the results of treating 48 patients with migraine, almost all of whom found they had complete or near complete relief of their symptoms after following his elimination diets. He, like many of the other doctors whose work followed, found that reactions to cereal grains were the most common problems.

In a more detailed study published in 1931, his book *Food Allergy, Its Manifestations, Diagnosis and Treatment,* he reported on a further 86 cases in much greater detail. The final results were that 73.1 per cent of the patients responded very well, 6.9 per cent had a fair response and 20 per cent had a poor response. In this trial he used a variety of dietary manoeuvres to sort out these patients, including cereal-free diets, rotary diversified diets and so forth.

In 1931 Dr R. M. Balyeat and Dr H. J. Rinkel assessed 202 migraine patients relying entirely on skin tests and *not* using elimination diets. In this trial they only obtained a 22 per cent excellent response rate and 38 per cent good response, confirming in general the superiority of elimination diets over skin testing. Also in 1931, the *Journal of Allergy* included a paper on allergic headache by Dr C. H. Eyerman. He had surveyed 63 patients using skin tests and elimination diets and obtained good results in 69 per cent of his cases.

In 1932 Dr E. L. de Gowin reported on 60 cases of migraine in the *Journal of Allergy*. After elimination diets, he claimed a success rate of 78 per cent.

In 1935, Dr J. M. Sheldon and Dr T. G. Randolph reported in the *American Journal of Medical Science*, their results of studying 127 migraine patients on elimination diets. They claimed a success rate of 60.8 per cent.

In 1937, Dr Albert Rowe reported a huge study of 247 patients assessed by a combination of skin tests and elimination diets. The success rate in this trial was 63.5 per cent good, 19.5 per cent fair and 17 per cent failure.

In 1952, Dr A. H. Unger and Dr L. Unger reported on their trial of elimination diets in the *Journal of Allergy*. They used elimination diets in 55 patients and found that 64 per cent responded excellently and 16 per cent had a good response.

In 1965, Dr R. S. Shapiro and Dr B. C. Eisenberg produced another paper on migraine and food allergy in the *Annals of Allergy*. These authors also used a combination of elimination diets and skin tests to diagnose their patients' allergies. In 100 patients they reported a 76 per cent success rate, of which 36 per cent became totally headache-free and 40 per cent noticed great improvement.

There have been several smaller trials in addition which, in the interests of brevity, I have not mentioned. Those using elimination diets essentially showed the same results as the trials that I have cited above. There is obviously some difficulty in categorizing success rates in migraine studies for obvious reasons. Most of the foods which are implicated are often difficult to avoid and patients vary a lot in their willingness to avoid foods to which they know they are sensitive. Thus, a patient whose allergies have been perfectly diagnosed may not come into the headache-free category purely because he is unwilling to avoid the foods causing his problems. Therefore, there must be a tendency to understate the potential benefit of this procedure. Of course, what the various authors are trying to prove is that food allergy causes migraine. The fact that some patients find it difficult to comply with the regime is irrelevant to proving this concept. As previously mentioned, techniques such as desensitization can help to get round this problem and therefore improve the results.

All of the above trials emanated from the United States of America and represented the position prior to 1979, when the first of the five British trials was published. If we compare the individual results relating to excellent or good improvement, the figures are as follows: Dr Albert Rowe in 1931 — 80 per cent; Dr E. de Gowin — 78 per cent; Dr Albert Rowe in 1937 — 83 per cent; Drs Unger and Unger — 80 per cent; Drs Shapiro and Eisenberg — 76 per cent; Drs Sheldon and Randolph — 60.8 per cent; Dr Eyerman — 69 per cent. It can be seen that five of these seven trials show a remarkable degree of consistency, all being close to 80 per cent successful. It must be remembered of course, that all these trials were carried out prior to there being any real knowledge of hydrocarbon sensitivity and before some aspects of food allergy such as masking had been completely appreciated.

Tyramine

For many years it has been well known that cheese, chocolate and red wine can often provoke migraine, and all these items contain an amino acid called tyramine. One theory that held sway for some time was that migraneurs were deficient in an enzyme called monoamine oxidase, an enzyme which we all possess and which is involved in metabolizing tyramine. However, deficiency of monoamine oxidase has only been reported during actual attacks, suggesting that it is a result of the problem rather than the cause of it. In addition, double-blind administration of tyramine to a number of patients who had improved on a low-tyramine diet failed to provoke migraine attacks. Thus, the reaction to these foods would seem to be more likely due to an allergy and when the huge variety of foods that can cause migraine is considered, this theory appears even more tenable. I am personally sure that these particular foods have become so well known as trigger factors because they are, on one hand, fairly common causes of migraine and, on the other hand, usually only eaten intermittently. Thus, bearing in mind the concept of masking, such items are more likely to be noticed as migraine precipitants than items such as milk or wheat, which are eaten daily.

The British Trials

We now come to three of the British trials, the first of which was published in May 1979 in *The Lancet*. The author was Dr Ellen Grant of the Department of Neurology at Charing Cross Hospital. Dr Grant had become interested in food allergy as a cause of migraine after visiting my clinic and, as I had already been investigating the subject for a few years, I advised her on the mechanisms of the elimination diet and so forth. Dr Grant had been very impressed at the number of contraceptive pill users and cigarette smokers who developed migraine and she discovered that getting patients to stop these practices had often resulted in distinct clinical improvements. She had also become convinced that many patients given ergotamine tartrate, the main specific anti-migraine drug, could become addicted to it. Eventually the drug itself could make the migraine problem worse because the patient had become possibly addicted and possibly allergic to it.

Before Dr Grant embarked on her trial of food allergy and

migraine, she had already discovered that if smokers stopped smoking and avoided items such as cheese, chocolate, citrus fruits, alcohol and other people's cigarette smoke, 53 per cent of them became free of their headaches. By avoiding the same foods and oral contraceptives 33 per cent of oral contraceptive users became headache-free too. Adopting the same restrictions and stopping ergotamine tartrate resulted in 13 per cent of the ergotamine users becoming headache-free. However, these success rates only indicate that these items are an important part of the overall problem, but not the whole part. Dr Grant therefore went ahead with a full food allergy study of 60 patients and 85 per cent of the patients became headache-free. Apart from asking patients to observe their reactions to individually-reintroduced foods, Dr Grant, like myself, advised the patients to monitor their pulse rates before taking their food, and again twenty minutes, forty minutes and sixty minutes after the food. Very frequently when a patient has a reaction there is a noticeable increase in pulse rate, usually over ten beats per minute, and this can help in the general assessment of whether the food is causing a reaction.

The bald statement that 85 per cent of patients became headache-free perhaps does not illustrate the degree of improvement as much as comparing the volume of drugs taken before the trial began and after. Before the trial, the patients involved in it took an average of 115 tablets a month, whether they were pain-killers, ergotamine tartrate or any other specific anti-migraine medication. After the trial an average of only 0.5 tablets a month were taken. I think it can be agreed that this is a startling reduction by any standard. Those who had been prescribed ergotamine tartrate had been taking approximately 1 mg per day, but all of them found they could do without this drug after the trial.

The second British trial of food allergy in migraine was published in July 1980 by *The Lancet*. The authors were Dr Jean Munro, Dr K. Zilka and Dr Claudio Carini of the National Hospital for Nervous Diseases and Dr Jonathon Brostoff of the Department of Immunology at the Middlesex Hospital Medical School. The trial was split into two main sections. In one part there was a standard elimination procedure followed by an attempt to corroborate the result of this procedure by the radioallergosorbent test (RAST test). In the first group 33 patients were studied and 23 of them did very well, giving a success rate of 70 per cent.

Another group of 26 patients were studied in which the RAST test was initially used diagnostically, followed by an elimination diet. This group did better and the success rate was recorded as being 88 per cent.

It is fair to state that the RAST test appears to be very useful in this trial, but this has never been found by any other investigators. It is possible that some refinements to the test which were introduced by Dr Brostoff made it a more useful tool.

Undoubtedly the most comprehensive trial of food allergy and migraine was published by *The Lancet* in October 1983. This trial was summarized as follows. Ninety-three per cent of 88 children with severe, frequent migraine recovered on low-risk allergy diets. The foods causing reactions were then identified by sequentially reintroducing these foods one at a time. The unique and totally convincing part of their trial was that the role of these foods in triggering the migraine was then corroborated by a huge series of double-blind studies of 40 of these patients. Anyone interested in the actual results of these double-blind studies can refer to the original papers, but here it will suffice to say that virtually all the children accurately reacted to the tins containing the foods to which they were known to be allergic. Neither the children who were receiving the specific tins of food nor the nurses who administered them knew what was in them. The placebo tins were indistinguishable in taste and texture from the tins containing the actual suspected food allergens. When an analysis of the results was performed, it was found that the statistical difference between the active and placebo tins was $p < 0.001$.

This double-blind assessment puts this trial way ahead of the previous trials in its validity. Most of the earlier trials, particularly the American ones, were carried out on fee-paying patients and for obvious reasons, it would be difficult to subject them to tests which would certainly cause a recurrence of their symptoms. In general, National Health Service patients are usually so grateful for the considerable time and expense which has been lavished on their case for no charge, that they are more than happy to subject themselves to additional testing after their problem has been elucidated, to further the cause of science. Private practitioners, working without the benefit of a grant have to face the formidable costs of making up all the placebo and active tin mixtures for double-blind study.

Secondary factors

For some years clinical ecologists and other allergists working with migraine patients have maintained that factors such as noise, bright lights, bangs on the head, travel, emotional upsets and exercise only act as a secondary factor in the production of migraine. These physicians, including myself, have basically observed that once a patient's allergies have been identified, these factors no longer seem to produce migraine. In other words, they seem to us to be factors which, when acting on a patient suffering from multiple allergies, seem to be 'the last straw that breaks the camel's back'. This view has received massive verification from this last trial, which found that before the diet thirteen patients reported that exercise could provoke their migraine, whereas after the trial only one patient found that this was the case.

Trauma of one sort or another, such as bangs on the head, was found to produce migraine in eleven of the patients prior to the trial, but only one after it. Ten patients considered that emotional factors triggered their migraine before the diet but none of them found this to be the case after the diet.

Travel was found to provoke migraine in nine patients prior to the diet but in none while on the diet. I am personally a little surprised at this finding because in my experience one of the main causes of migraine caused by travel is petrol or diesel fumes and these were presumably still present after the diet. This finding is, in fact, the only one in the whole trial which conflicts with my clinical experience.

Bright lights, heat and noise were found to be much less likely to provoke migraine while patients were on the low-risk diet. Very significantly, perfumes and/or cigarette smoke proved problems in ten patients before the diet commenced and continued to do so for nine of them while on the low risk diet. In other words, as intimated earlier, these hydrocarbon exposures are primary excitants and must be included in the basic evaluation of the patient.

As Dr Grant noticed, 'chemicals in the home environment can make this testing difficult for out-patients'. The whole topic of chemicals in foods, and indoor and outdoor air pollution has been discussed earlier and when these factors are taken into account success rates in dealing with migraine patients improve considerably.

As mentioned earlier, editors of medical journals like to take papers concentrating on one particular factor such as food allergy. To those who work in the subject, it is known that hydrocarbon sensitivity plays a very large role in some patients and in other patients intestinal candidiasis can be very important. I would like to see in the very near future a trial in which the physician can use a food allergy work-up combined with a hydrocarbon work-up and taking into account intestinal candidiasis. From my own experience I am sure that the results would be even better than those obtained already and taking these other factors into account would reduce the failure rate dramatically.

Associated symptoms
Another major fact to emerge from these trials, is that a high proportion of patients have many other associated symptoms, and furthermore, that when they are placed on a safe diet that these symptoms disappear at the same time as the migraine.

Dr Theron Randolph, the father of clinical ecology, has always maintained that looking at one disease entity by itself is a fundamental mistake. It has led to over-specialization, false pigeon-holing and to doctors being unable to 'see the wood for the trees'. In fact, logically, I should not be writing this book on a single disease entity such as migraine. Dr Randolph regards migraine, for example, as just one symptom caused by food and/or environmental allergy amongst a number of other symptoms. In this view I agree with him, but for the time being, as most physicians and patients think a condition like migraine as a separate disease entity, it is helpful for migraine trials and books like this to bridge the gap between this new thinking and the traditional view of disease.

Dr Grant noted that very many of her patients had symptoms such as lethargy, anxiety, depression, abdominal pain, constipation, diarrhoea, dizziness, painful periods, obesity, breast lumps and recurring cystitis. The attacks of recurring cystitis were not usually accompanied by any evidence of bacterial infection. Most of these symptoms cleared at the same time as the migraine and recurred when specific foods were reintroduced into the diet. The most dramatic discovery of all, however, related to those patients who also had blood-pressure problems. Fifteen out of 60 patients in Dr Grant's trial suffered with high blood-pressure as well as migraine before the trial but afterwards it was found that in all cases their blood-pressure had dropped to within the normal range and they no longer needed to take blood pressure medications. Many other physicians have noted similar responses, and as blood-pressure is one of the major influences on human health, the implications of this are hard to exaggerate.

Professor Soothill's trial at Great Ormond Street also has enormous implications in terms of associated symptoms. Of the 88 children in the trial, 61 had abdominal pain, diarrhoea and flatulence before the diet, but only 8 continued to have these symptoms while on the diet. Forty-one of the children also had behavioural disorders before the trial commenced and only 5 still had problems while they were on the diet. This supports the view of many doctors who have worked on the theory that hyperactivity in children is usually caused by allergies to food or food additives. Most of the behavioural disorders in this trial were of a hyperkinetic variety. In other words, these children were mostly suffering from what is called hyperactivity. This type of problem is very widespread these days and appears to be becoming more prevalent. The Hyperactive Children's Support Group has a vast number of members and have collected details of thousands of children who have found relief after eliminating certain foods or additives from their diets. In addition, several authors like Dr Doris Rapp of Buffalo in the United States of America, have written extensively on this subject. Professor Soothill's trial lends enormous credence to their work. Aches in the limb were also noted in 41 patients and this symptom disappeared in all but five by the time they had been on the trial for some days. Amongst the 88 children on the trial, 14 also suffered from epileptic fits. While on the diet only two of them had this problem and the other twelve were able to discontinue their anti-epileptic drugs. They only had a recurrence of their fits if they slipped up on their diet. The same team that did the original trial on migraine are now proceeding with a trial of a large number of epileptic patients to try and further verify this finding, which is also of course of enormous significance.

Persistent rhinitis (runny nose) occurred in 34 of these

children and this reduced to 15 during the diet. Of course, inhalant allergies such as house dust, house-dust mite and mould are well-known causes of this complaint and it is now becoming recognized that food allergies are the cause in many patients where there is no evidence of inhalant allergy. I wrote a paper for *The Practitioner* (August 1983 edition) describing how food and inhalant allergies can be identified in this chronic and unpleasant condition.

Recurring mouth ulcers, a complaint that has always mystified the medical profession, were present in fifteen cases before the diet and in only two cases after it.

Persistent vaginal discharge reduced from a total of eleven cases prior to the diet to one case afterwards.

Asthma, which like rhinitis is a condition known in many cases to be caused by inhaled allergies, reduced from seven cases pre-diet to three cases while on the diet.

Finally, eczema reduced from six cases before the diet to three while on it.

All these symptoms recurred with the same reliability as the migraine on the double-blind trials but, of course, because there were not, for example, as many epileptic cases as migraine patients, the statistical significance in these particular conditions would be lower. However, in the case of abdominal pain, behavioural disorders and the limb pain problems, the numbers were so large (all over 40) that the statistical significance of the results is clearly high.

This trial, therefore, clearly demonstrates that food allergy is a very important factor in migraine and certainly in these children would appear to cause nearly the whole problem. It also demonstrates that food allergy can cause a great number of other major illnesses.

In September 1984 a further trial was published in *The Lancet*. This trial was boldly titled, 'Migraine *is* a food-allergic disease.' The authors were again Dr Jean Monro, Dr Jonathan Brostoff and Dr Claudio Carini. This study was performed on nine patients with severe migraine. After the usual elimination diet procedure the allergenic foods were then fed to the patients again, either with sodium cromoglycate (Nalcrom) or with a placebo. In the patients who were fed the active food and the placebo, immune complexes were produced, followed by symptoms. In those who were fed the active food complex and sodium cromoglycate, no reaction and no immune complexes were discovered. This demonstrated that the food-allergic reaction is the actual cause of migraine and not just a precipitating factor. It also proved that, for a single meal, sodium cromoglymate could exert a protective effect, both in stopping the formation of immune complexes and in preventing symptoms. Unfortunately, in clinical experience this protective effect appears to be very short-lived and in practice Nalcrom appears useful only for protection against the occasional isolated meal. Its use on a more continual basis is exceptionally disappointing.

In October 1984 Dr Brostoff was again involved in a trial, this time reported in *Clinical Allergy*. The subject was abdominal migraine and food senstivity in children. His colleagues were Dr D. Bentley and Dr Adriana Catchburian of Ealing Hospital in Southall. Abdominal migraine is a condition characterized by recurring abdominal pain, nausea and vomiting. In addition, all the patients in this particular trial had a family history of classical migraine. As a result of selective withdrawal of the most suspected foods, ten out of the twelve children in the trial became either free of symptoms or had very reduced symptoms. The authors concluded that abdominal migraine in children was associated with food sensitivity and that the RAST test (in children at least) was of no use in defining the implicated foods.

There has been an enormous amount of work which has demonstrated that food allergy is the major cause of migraine. It should be noted that no trial following the principles we have mentioned has failed to demonstrate a positive correlation of food allergy with migraine.

13.

THE ROOTS OF ALLERGY

Why does allergy develop? What do we currently know of this and, if we can draw some conclusions from work on the subject, might we be able to prevent the occurrence of migraine and other similar allergic disorders? Over the past forty years, several major factors have come to light. To those practitioners who are dealing with patients on an everyday basis, these factors are becoming more and more valid as patients seem to respond to measures suggested by the concepts I am just about to discuss. The main factors at the root of the allergic problem appear to be: (1) Basic nutritional deficiencies; (2) A monotonous repetitive diet of foods recently introduced into the human diet; (3) The chemical adulteration of food; (4) Chronic intestinal thrush (candidiasis). This list is not in order of importance as, in fact, I think that the chronic intestinal thrush is possibly the most important factor.

In discussing these factors, I must emphasize that we have nowhere near the weight of documentary evidence to support these ideas that, for example, we have to support the concept that food allergy is the major cause of migraine. Approximately seven years ago, many physicians knew from their daily experience that food allergens could cause migraine. However, it took many years to prove it to the extent that we have now. We are roughly in the same position now with the factors I am about to discuss. That is not to say, however, that we have no documentary proof, because we have. The effect that basic nutritional factors could have on animals (and hence man) was most brilliantly demonstrated in 1945 by what has been known as the Pottenger Cat Studies.

The Pottenger Cat Studies

Drug companies are well aware that in most respects cats respond similarly to human beings and so they are widely used for testing drugs. These experiments were suggested by Pottenger's observation that cats fed on a raw meat and raw milk diet were much better operative risks than those fed cooked meat and raw milk. In a series of experiments, one group of cats was fed on a diet of two-thirds *raw* meat, one-third raw milk and cod-liver oil. A second group was fed on a diet of two-thirds *cooked* meat, one-third raw milk and cod-liver oil. Nine hundred cats were studied over a period of ten years.

The cats receiving raw meat and raw milk reproduced normally, had few abortions, nursed their young well, had very good behaviour patterns and a high resistance to infections and parasites.

The cats receiving the cooked meat reproduced poorly in general and there was an abortion rate of 25 per cent in the first generation, increasing to 70 per cent in the second generation. Many cats died in labour and the mortality rate in the kittens was high. The cats were irritable and difficult to handle, *skin lesions and allergies* were frequent and became progressively worse from generation to generation while the cats remained on the same diet. In addition, the oral arches narrowed, and osteomyelitis, cardiac lesions, thyroid disease, nephritis, hepatitis, arthritis and many other conditions familiar to human beings all became common. Of the cats maintained entirely on the cooked meat/raw milk diet, the kittens of the third generation were so degenerated that none of them survived the first six months of life, thereby terminating the strain.

Cats of this first and second generation cooked-meat group were later returned to a raw-meat diet. Of enormous significance was the fact that it took three to four generations before the offspring regained good health. In the beginning of this century, people in the Western world started to eat highly refined and processed foods, with a high percentage of our food cooked. We are, therefore, in approximately the third or fourth generations of eating such foods and increasingly we are getting the same diseases that the cats did.

There follows from this work the enormous implication that a condition which may be currently considered genetic in origin could originally stem from poor nutrition in an earlier generation. The other less happy implication is that really adequate nutrition may fail to correct chronic diseases within one generation which are already occurring in that generation. This is not to say, however, that allergy management could not do the same job.

The aforementioned trial is not a plea for human beings to exist entirely on raw food and milk. It is, however, a demonstration that inadequate nutrition can have a disastrous effect in terms of disease on one species and that there is no reason to believe that inadequate diet could not have the same effect on human beings. Pottenger surmised that the specific problem could well be the denaturing of protein by heat. Certainly, heating meat alters its physiochemical state in the same way as processing other foods will alter their ability to remain perfect for the maintenance of health.

Basic Nutritional Deficiencies
In the past few years there has been an enormous upsurge in interest in the nutritional basis of disturbances of the whole immune system. There is no question that the immune system is involved with the engendering of migraine and there is now no doubt that deficiencies or excesses of certain nutrients can have the most dramatic effects on the proper functioning of the whole immune system. Perhaps one of the best single surveys of this subject was published in the *Journal of the American Medical Association* in January 1981, entitled, 'Single Nutrient Effects on Immunological Functions.' It was a report of a workshop sponsored by the Department of Food and Nutrition and the Nutrition Advisory Group of the American Medical Association. In the summary of this workshop several major statements summarized the work of enormous numbers of investigators in this subject. What follows for the next few pages I am afraid requires a minor knowledge of immunology to fully understand. Perhaps readers who are totally unacquainted with immunologic phenomena will excuse me, but I am including this information partly to complete the background to this subject and partly to give lay readers a flavour of the wealth of information supporting the concept that adequate diet is essential to proper immune function.

The summary of this report stated that immune system dysfunction can result from single nutrient deficiencies or excesses alone or in combination with generalized protein/energy malnutrition. Acquired immune dysfunctions in man occur with deficiencies of iron, zinc, vitamins A and B_{12}, pyridoxine and folic acid and with excesses of essential fatty acids and vitamin E. Additional micronutrients are important for maintaining immunologic competence in animals. Deficits or excesses of many trace elements and single nutrients thus have potential for causing immune dysfunctions in man. Since nutritionally-induced immune dysfunction is generally reversible, it is important to recognize and identify clinical illnesses in which immunologic dysfunctions are of nutritional origin. Correction of malnutrition should lead to prompt reversal of acquired immune dysfunctions.

Vitamins

Perhaps the most important immunological effects produced by vitamins stem from deficiencies in the B group, especially with deficiencies of pyridoxine, pantothenic acid, folic acid and vitamin B_{12}. The other B vitamins have very little direct effect on the immune system. A defiency of pyridoxine depresses cellular and humoral immunity in animals. Deficiency of pantothenic acid appears to inhibit the stimulation of antibody-producing cells and their ability to produce new immunoglobulins. Folic acid deficiency leads to patients having an impaired ability to respond to skin testing.

Vitamin C appears to influence the ability of the phagocytic cells to perform their germ-killing functions and to promote wound healing. Vitamin A deficiency in animals leads to depletion of thymic lymphoctyes and depressed lymphocytic response to certain stimulants. Vitamin E deficiency depresses the immunologic response to antigens and has other similar effects. In dosage above the average, vitamin E seems to exert many beneficial effects on the immune system, but in very high dosage it has an inhibitory effect on many immune functions.

Minerals

The most important minerals in terms of the immune system appear to be iron, zinc and selenium. Iron deficiency, which is often seen as an isolated nutritional problem, causes immune dysfunction is huge numbers of patients. These patients demonstrate impaired skin hypersensitivity and very poor macrophage and neutrophil functions. There is no doubt at all that the immune system is extremely sensitive to iron availability and will adversely respond to deficiencies that are so small that they do not even cause iron deficiency anaemia. Conversely, excessive iron can be deleterious and can saturate plasma iron-binding proteins. This in turn can increase the availability of iron for uptake by various micro-organisms which in turn may lead to sepsis. Zinc deficiency produces abnormalities in both cellular and humoral immunity. Lymphocytes demonstrate a decreased response to certain stimulants and T-killer cell activity. An increase in dietary selenium, either alone or in combination with vitamin E, appears to enhance immune responsiveness to vaccine antigens in animals.

Fatty Acids

This is an area in which there is much current exciting research. In the report we have been discussing it was noted that a deficiency of essential fatty acids depresses both primary and secondary antibody responses to both T-cell dependent and independent antigens in mice. At the time of this report a similar effect had not been reported in man. On the other hand, excess polyunsaturated fatty acids produce widespread immunologic defects in laboratory animals.

It has been one of the greatest oversights by the medical profession in general to assume that most of the population have nutritionally adequate diets from which they acquire the optimum amount of all the minerals, vitamins and essential fatty acids etc. that they need. For a start, patients' individual needs vary greatly and, furthermore, the enormous switch which has occurred this century from naturally-occurring foods to pre-packaged manufactured foods has taken little account of the human need for many of these micronutrients.

Work such as I have briefly outlined is now going on at many laboratories throughout the world and hundreds of papers are produced annually on this subject. In this book it is inappropriate to go into much more detail, but one of the best books devoted to this subject is called *Nutrition Against Disease*, by Roger J. Williams, who is emeritus professor of chemistry at the University of Texas.

In Great Britain we have recently seen the setting up of the British Society for Nutritional Medicine and there are now a number of physicians and laboratories in this country busily identifying the nutritional status of individual patients. Once this has been done measures can be taken to correct the deficiencies or excesses that are discovered. The laboratories can identify these problems by blood serum, hair analysis and sweat test examinations, amongst others. It is my practice to refer for analysis migraine patients who from preliminary investigation appear to have widespread immune dysfunction.

2. A Monotonous, Repetitive Diet of Foods Recently Introduced into the Human Diet

Mankind has eaten vegetables, fruit, fish and meat since the Stone Age. Physicians working with food-allergic patients know that these foods, especially in their organic form, are for most patients the safest. The reason for this probably is that we have, as a species, eaten these foods for two to three million years and we are hence fairly well adapted to them. Any of our forebears who could not tolerate these types of food have probably tended to die out. The Stone Age diet was conceived by Dr Richard Mackarness as a relatively safe diet on which many food-allergic patients would improve as it avoided all the common food allergens. A perusal of the common foods implicated with migraine as indicated by the last food trials shows wheat to be the commonest item found. Corn, milk, eggs, cane and beet sugar, yeast and soya-beans are also amongst the more common offenders, although it is to be noted that orange, which of course is a fruit, is also a common cause of migraine.

Although bread is regarded by many people to be the 'staff of life', most people are surprised to learn that cereals such as wheat and corn are a relatively recent addition to the human diet. Corn was originally planted in Egypt 4,000 years ago, but there is no evidence of cereals being grown in Great Britain prior to the Roman invasion around 2,000 years ago. Yeast has probably been used for about 8,000 years, originally to make scrumpy. Sugar was unknown in Great Britain until cane sugar was brought from the West Indies in the sixteenth century, only about 400 years ago.

Soya-beans have been introduced into this country only since 1955. They now crop up in our diet in a multitude of ways, usually in the form of soya-bean oil or soya-bean flour. Soya-bean oil is found in many wholemeal breads. It is also present, usually vaguely labelled as vegetable oil, in margarine, ice cream, salad dressings and mayonnaise. Soya bean flour is also found in sausages, luncheon meats and confectionery. Thus, most of our major foods have only been in our diet for a couple of hundred — or thousand — years and, in terms of evolution and adaptation, two thousand years is only yesterday. In the chapter on the elimination diet, I detailed the multitude of ways in which corn creeps into most people's everyday diet. Many people eat corn in over ten different ways every day of their life. The invention of complex food mixtures by the food industry has made it very easy to eat small amounts of wheat, corn, milk, eggs, soy, cane and beet sugar very frequently throughout the day. It would appear that this frequent 'peppering' of our enzyme systems by these foods is very important in the engendering of food sensitivity.

Part of the evidence for this is that it very frequently turns out that foods which the patient eats most frequently and addictively are the ones to which he turns out to be sensitive. Admittedly, by the time the patient is seen by the doctor, the addictive factor may be due to the allergy having developed.

Further evidence is provided by observations related to the development of tolerance to foods that at one time produced allergy. If an allergic food is left out of the diet for a period of between three months and two years, tolerance will develop in most instances. It is then observed that if the food is only eaten about once every four or five days, then this tolerance will be maintained. If the food is eaten more frequently, the tolerance is usually destroyed and an allergic response will again result. These observations are the basis of the rotation diet, which is often useful in the management of patients with food allergies. The idea of such a diet is that no food is repeated more than once every four or five days. On such a diet, new food allergies virtually never occur, but it is of course difficult to maintain socially. Nevertheless, the effectiveness of such regimes is further proof that the frequency with which a food is ingested is very important in the causation of allergy.

3. Chemicals in Food and the Environment

That chemicals can lead to allergic phenomena has already been described in the chapter on chemical susceptibility. Chemicals are known not to be antigenic, but it is thought that some

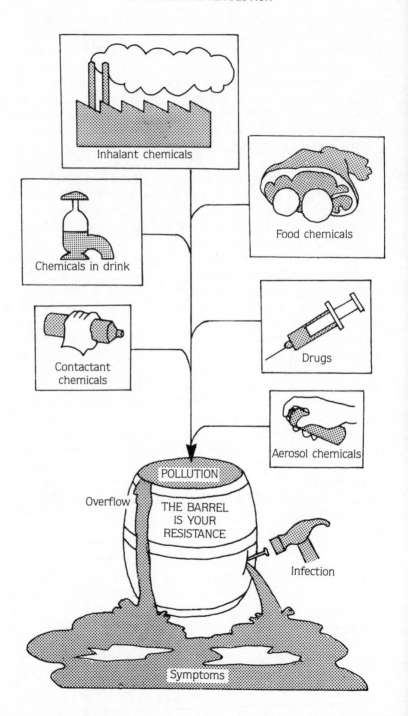

bind to proteins to form haptens (incomplete antigens). There is evidence to suggest furthermore that chemicals can contribute to making the mucous membranes of the intestines leaky. I will go into this in greater detail later in connection with intestinal candidiasis. In addition, it is likely that chemicals can lead to food susceptibility in terms of the total load they create on the immune system. Dr William Rea of the Brookhaven Medical Centre in Dallas recently invented the barrel concept of allergy.

This illustrates the concept that various allergies can have a summative effect, and when enough of this effect occurs, the barrel overflows and symptoms result. In my experience, I have seen many patients who will react to certain foods when in a polluted environment, but not when in a clean environment.

4. Chronic Intestinal Thrush (Candidiasis)

This whole subject has already been discussed in Chapter 7. Here it is only described in the context in which it may dovetail with other basic causes of allergy. It will be recalled tht in the chapter on chronic intestinal candidiasis I described how the mycelia of the fungal form of Candida can penetrate the mucous membrane of the digestive tract, leading to a leaky mucous membrane. A few years ago an article in *The Lancet*, abstracted later in the Society for Clinical Ecology Newsletter, covered a controlled study indicating that patients with food or skin allergies had leaky mucous membranes which could admit many more protein molecules than was normal. Patients with multiple food and chemical sensitivities thus became that way because antibodies were formed to the antigenic proteins in food, pollens and even their own microbiological flora of the gut. This flora includes fungi, such as Candida, trichophyton and epidermophyton. As stated earlier, mucous membranes can also be made to leak by excessive exposure to toxic chemicals and almost certainly by the sort of nutritional deficiencies which have been described earlier in this chapter. Thus, the critical mechanisms underlying the whole food and chemical allergy problem are probably related to leaky mucous membranes in the intestine and these are in turn caused by the various factors which have been discussed in this chapter. Some of these factors may be more important in some patients and others may be more important in others. I have the opinion myself, based on general experience of dealing with patients rather than hard clinical data, that the Candida problem is probably the most significant. Very likely in many patients these factors interweave to produce the final result. Quite probably, once the situation occurs in which the development of food sensitivity is likely, repeated ingestion of a certain food which is new to our diet will then make it further likely that an allergy will develop.

Resistance and Adaptation

Up to now we have talked almost exclusively about the various factors that constitute the insult to the host, that is, the patient. Like all equations, however, the final result depends on the interplay of two factors: (1) the nature of the insult or attack on the host; (2) the resistance and natural adaptive resources of the host.

The work that has most clarified this aspect was done by Hans Selye, the eminent physiologist, working in his laboratory at the University of Montreal. Selye's work on what is termed 'the general adaptation syndrome' will almost certainly eventually rank amongst the greatest medical discoveries of all time. He has basically clarified the mechanisms of adaptation to stress. By stress I do not just mean psychological stress but also and, more importantly, the struggle of the human body to stay healthy in the face of the whole gamut of potentially harmful agents with which it is in daily contact. Selye has defined stress as the rate at which wear and tear is induced in the body by the whole process of living. It is now known that cortisone, which is produced by the cortex of our adrenal glands, is our main defence against allergic reactions of all types. Selye was the first to demonstrate that cortisone had a protective effect and was also able to mobilize the body's other defences against allergic reactions and other harmful events. In 1936 Selye published a letter in the journal *Nature* entitled, 'A Syndrome Produced by Diverse Nocuous Agents.' The letter started as follows, 'Experiments on rats show that, if the organism is severely damaged by acute, non-specific noxious agents, such as exposure to cold, surgical injury, excessive muscular exercise or intoxications with sublethal doses of diverse drugs, a typical syndrome appears, the symptoms of which are independent of the nature of the damaging agent or the pharmacological type of drug employed and represents rather a response to damage as such.' Later in the letter he described the three stages of the general adaptation syndrome. Stage 1 (the alarm reaction) started about six to forty-eight hours after the initial injury. It is akin to what most doctors refer to as surgical shock and is characterized by low blood-pressure, loss of muscle tone and shrinkage of the adrenal glands as they pump out as much cortisone as possible. There were also other symptoms, such as leakage of fluid from the smaller blood vessels into the surrounding tissues.

Stage 2 started about forty-eight hours after the original injury. There was now considerable enlargement of the adrenal glands and the swelling in the tissues produced by the leakage of fluid from the blood vessels started to subside. The pituitary gland, which controls virtually all the other glands in the body, produced increased amounts of a hormone (adreno-cortico-stimulating hormone) which in turn caused the adrenal glands to produce more cortisone.

When further small repeated doses of the harmful stimulus were given, be it an allergy-producing stimulus or any other stimulus, the rats built up a resistance. Hence they had become adapted and in this phase they outwardly showed no symptoms at all.

If the rats in this adapted stage were removed from the harmful stress, for example the persistent cold stimulus, it was found that they lost their newly-acquired resistance to the cold within a few days. When reintroduced to the cold environment again they had to go through the Stage 1 alarm reaction. Conversely, if the rats were left in the cold, they continued adapting for a long time, apparently having grown completely used to it.

This is of course exactly what has been described earlier in the book in Chapter 2, when we were talking of masking to foods. This mechanism of masking represents the continued application of the harmful stimulus and the body's adapted response to it. We also noted the exaggerated adverse response (Rinkel's hyperacute response) when the body was re-exposed to that food after a period (five days plus) of avoiding it. In other words, Rinkel's hyperacute response is a Stage 1 alarm reaction.

If the rats continued to be exposed for a long time to the cold stimulus they seemed at first to be perfectly well, but after a period of time they became ill and eventually died. They had entered a stage of maladaption and eventually a stage of exhaustion. The symptoms in this Stage 3 (maladaption and then exhaustion) were similar to Stage 1 (the alarm stage). In Stage 3 only complete removal from the harmful stimulus would produce a healthy animal. The transition from the adapted to the maladapted/exhaustion stage is clinically known as the start of the current illness.

Why patients go from the adapted phase to the non-adapted phase is not always obvious. In some patients there appears to be no particular reason why their migraines should start at a particular age. Maybe their body is just becoming older and less able to keep up their successful adaptation. In other cases it appears obvious that 'the straw that broke the camel's back' was an event that produced a temporary excessive stress on the patient's system. In many patients migraine problems start soon after a severe attack of flu, glandular fever or a similar virus illness. Childbirth, major operations and accidents are physically stressful events which can also be the 'final straw'. Major psychological stresses can also have the same effect. In a recent study published in the United States of America it was shown that bereavement caused a diminution in the T-lymphocyte count in most patients. The level of the T-lymphocytes is possibly one of the better indications of the competence of the immune system to deal with allergic phenomena.

There is a condition called 'royal free disease', which is a severe meningitis-like illness. In a high proportion of patients, after they recover from the primary illness they are never the same again. Many suffer from a whole range of symptoms like fatigue, depression, headaches, nausea and so on. I have treated a lot of these patients and most of these symptoms are related to food allergy and can be eradicated by eliminating their food allergies. I am sure, therefore, that in these patients the severe viral illness was just a major stressful event which caused these patients to start to react to dormant food allergies.

Thus, people start to react to foods in the middle part of their lives due to their failure to maintain their adaptation to them. Foods which had appeared to be perfectly innocuous for often twenty to forty years suddenly become harmful. The whole root of the migraine problem can thus be summarized by the diagram shown opposite:

Although everything in this diagram is I think basically valid

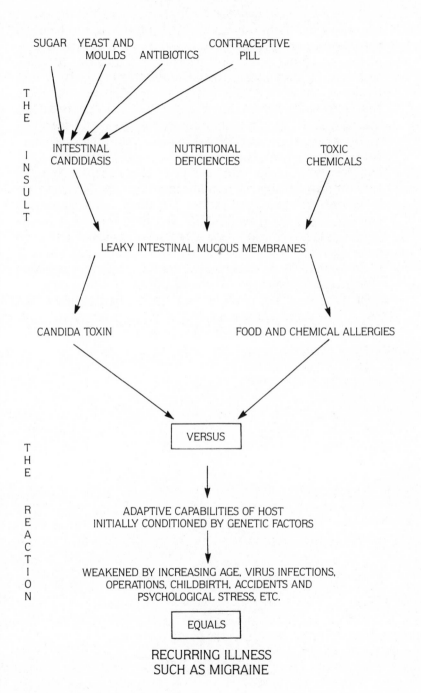

and there is much evidence to support it, there is an awful lot that we still do not know. Most problems can have an explanation at various levels. I have sought to explain this disease in terms of the insulting factors and the adaptive reactions of the patient to these aggravating factors. This might be described as the macroreaction. The microreaction, that is the particulars of the cellular or immunological response, are not at all well understood at the present time. The immunologic reaction to most foods is as yet totally unknown. Although a few food reactions are modulated by immunoglobulin E (IgE) the vast majority are not. It is thought that immunoglobulin G, perhaps IgG 4, may be the one that is involved in most food-allergic reactions, but this is pure speculation at the moment. The fact that we do not as yet understand the immunological response, however, does not mean that we cannot adequately deal with the condition. It could well be fifty years before the details of the immunological response are finally identified. In the meantime, there are millions of migraine patients who can be helped and often completely cured by the knowledge that is currently available.

14

ACCEPTING THESE CONCEPTS

The non-medical reader may at this point be inclined to wonder, 'why with this volume of evidence is this approach not already generally accepted throughout the medical profession? Furthermore, how long will it take to become so?' As many people have asked me in the past, when will this become available on the National Health Service? The answer to this question is when the medical establishment fully accepts this approach as valid.

I was once discussing with Dr Dale Peters, a very eminent American psychiatrist and clinical ecologist, my observation that patients seem to see the sense in the clinical ecology approach to illness much quicker than doctors. He made the perceptive remark, 'Well Dr Mansfield, you must appreciate that patients do not have the disadvantage of a medical education.' To fully understand this remark, it must be remembered that for well over two thousand years the history of medicine has demonstrated a constant schism between the two main directions of medical thought and philosophy.

One direction of medical thought can best be described as the rationalist school, and at the moment this school of thought dominates the teaching at medical schools throughout most of the world. This school prefers the approach of knowledge derived from the study of pathology (the study of organs, blood, etc.) followed by symptom suppression, for example by the use of drugs. The other direction is the empirical school of thought. This approach is based on the observation of the patient's symptoms and his inter-reaction with his environment, using the term in its widest sense. The approach described in this book is, of course, of the empirical school.

Throughout medical history these two main currents of

thought have flowed their separate courses, which have conflicted and yet have exerted influences on each other. There are some examples of empirical thought in rationalist teaching and vice versa. Certainly the rationalist approach has brought about many major advances in medicine, but the biggest advance of all, the GERM concept of disease was initially an empirical idea which was strongly resisted for many years by the medical establishment of the day. Bacteria and viruses are of course external environmental agents and their effect on human beings is now well accepted.

There now follows a list of the main physicians and scientists who have had the most influence on the rationalist and empirical schools of thought. It is interesting to note that between 200 AD and 1500 AD the rationalist school of thought held total sway, with no one advocating empirical thought at all.

Empirical	Rationalist
Hippocrates (c.460-c.357 BC)	Aristotle (384-322 BC)
Celsus (about 100)	Praxagoras, Erasistratos
Sextus Empiricus (about 200)	Galen (c.130-c.200)
Paracelsus (1493-1541)	Descartes (1596-1650)
J. B. VanHelmont (1578-1644)	Thomas Willis (1622-1675
Francis Bacon (1561-1626)	Hermann Boerhaave (1668-1738)
Thomas Sydenham (1624-1689)	William Cullen (1710-1790)
Giorgio Baglivi (1668-1707)	John Brown (1755-1788)
Georg Ernst Stahl (1660-1734)	Benjamin Rush (1745-1813)
Philippe Pinel (1745-1826)	Xavier Bichat (1771-1802)
Samuel Hahnemann (1755-1843)	F. J. V. Broussais (1772-1838)
Rene Laennec (1781-1826)	Claude Bernard (1813-1878)
Constantine Hering (1800-1880)	Rudolf Virchow (1821-1902)
Oliver Wendell Holmes (1809-1894)	Abraham Flexner (about 1900)

Sir Francis Bacon, who was a founder of modern science and an empiricist, believed that the purpose of science was to observe, describe and characterize the processes of nature, rather than necessarily to explain them. Hippocrates made the empirical observation that certain people were harmed by eating cheese, but most are not. Therefore there must be something in the reactivity of the individual rather than in the cheese itself. This conflicted with a tendency of most physicians of the rationalist school initiated by Aristotle to prefer pathological knowledge over symptomatic observations, ignoring symptoms unless they happened to fit in with their preconceived concepts.

Very typical of the rationalist thought process is the quote from Aristotle himself, 'We suppose scientists to be wiser than men of experience . . . and this is because the former know the cause, but the latter do not. For men of experience know that the thing is so, but do not know why, while the others know the why and the cause.' *It would be fine if they did, but they do not.*

This attitude, particularly in regard to medicine, reveals the most amazing scientific conceit. Scientists are nowhere near explaining, for example, the various chemical and immunological phenomena related to most chronic disease processes. The direction of most research in the rationalist-dominated medical schools is in the reporting of 'objective' findings from laboratory experiments. The *British Medical Journal* is full of reports of the 'serum rhubarb' findings, as they are irreverently referred to by many disenchanted physicians. Doctors reading these papers are usually as a loss to see how they can possibly relate to their daily problems with patients. Such papers are, however, respectable research and are an essential prerequisite for a young physician climbing the academic tree in a rationalist-dominated medical world. Papers reporting empirical research, even with such safeguards as double-blind trials, are not respectable in a relationalist-dominated medical society. Any aspiring young physician would be warned off such research by his elders and betters. Perhaps, though, the most fundamental difference between the two schools of thought is a spiritual one and this is therefore tied up with basic differences in human nature.

- Rationalists regard the scientific intellect as supreme.
- Empiricists tend to be less impressed with man's intellect, more religious and more interested in their common humanity with their patients.
- The function of empiricism is curative.
- The function of rationalism is to explain.
- Empiricism is orientated to the needs of the patient.
- Rationalism is often more orientated to the needs of the physician.

My rationalist medical school education taught me to focus my attention on to specific disease entities and on pathological findings, especially objective laboratory findings. It was necessary to find something wrong with the patient with objective tests in order to have a 'rational basis for treatment'.

The treatment then took the direction of opposing, combating or suppressing symptoms with analgesic drugs, anti-spasmodic drugs, anti-inflammatory drugs, anti-arthritic drugs and so on.

In the last century Constantine Hering taught that the suppression of acute illness tends to promote chronic illness. He also taught that the natural processes of healing functioned best when the physician promoted the reversion of chronic symptoms to acute symptoms. In this respect Hering foresaw the basic concept of clinical ecology; that a return to health requires an initial clearing of the chronic adaptive state (as, for example, on the five- to six-day hypoallergenic diet) after which time chronic symptoms can revert to acute symptoms (Rinkel's hyperacute response). At this stage the various excitants can be identified.

Many unfortunate things result from the preoccupation with pathology which characterizes the majority of present-day physicians.

Firstly, if a physician cannot find anything objectively wrong, he may not know what to do for his patient other than to reassure him or send him to a psychiatrist. In the case of migraine and other similar related disorders, there are virtually never any objective findings and migraneurs are frequently regarded by the medical profession as neurotics. Rheumatoid arthritis, for example, which is a condition replete with objective pathological laboratory findings, is a much more 'medically respectable' disease.

Most physicians, because of the training which focuses their attention, belief and behaviour on the rationalist approach, find it difficult to accept empirical approaches and regard them as unscientific or not being within the scope of the practice of medicine. An example of this is the role of cigarette smoking in the causation of lung cancer, a classic instance of an environmental stimulus causing a disease process. In 1958 I was a medical student and, having reviewed all the clinical papers supporting this view, I discussed the matter with several consultants at my medical school. In view of the weight of evidence I wanted to know why the fact that cigarette-smoking was a cause of lung cancer was not at that time being taught at my medical school. I was told that, if I believed that cigarette smoking was a cause of lung cancer, I was mad. That lung cancer could be caused by an environmental agent, such as a simple cigarette, was beyond belief. These physicians were much more interested in teaching the various histological forms that cancer could take rather than the environmental agents that could cause it. Of course nowadays this idea is almost totally accepted, but it has only been due to about thirty years of constant bludgeoning with more and more facts that this has been achieved. One of the interesting things about medicine is that it is often hard to establish the specific time that a new concept became generally acceptable. In which year, for example, was it finally accepted that cigarette smoking was the main cause of lung cancer? Possibly about five years ago, as I do not remember any concerted arguments to the contrary being advanced in the last five years. This is, in truth, no particular point in time. As Dr Ronald Finn once told me, there are four stages in the development of the new medical idea:

Stage 1:   You are mad.
Stage 2:   I suppose there might be something in it.
Stage 3:   There could be something in it, but where is the proof?
Stage 4:   Well, of course we knew all along.

Dr Finn thinks that we are in Stage 3 at the moment in regard to the clinical ecologic view of medicine. However, because of all these conflicting outlooks, it may be quite a long time before this approach is available in all clinics and hospitals, despite the positive evidence we have. There is no disadvantage in terms of cost in this approach to migraine, as it is indeed highly cost-effective. Four or five consultations and couple of skin-testing sessions will often obviate the need for repeated consultations extending over twenty or more years and constant drugging with pain-killing drugs and migraine preventives. There is also, of course, the enormous economic advantage of patients who suffer from migraine no longer having to take extensive time off work or working frequently well below their par.

I would like to thank Dr Karl Humiston of New York for much of the source material for this chapter.

15.

SUMMARY AND CONCLUSION

In this book I have described the underlying primary causes of migraine and methods for dealing with these underlying causes. Precipitants, such as tension, flashing lights, blows to the head, exercise and so on are secondary and cause no problems once the primary causes have been eliminated.

Food allergy plays the greatest single part in the causation of this disease. The foods involved are quite diverse and foods that in the past were thought to be the most important precipitants, such as cheese and chocolate, are not in fact the most common offenders. The most frequent offenders are in fact day-to-day foods like wheat, corn, milk, sugars, orange and so on.

The concepts of food addiction and masking are vital to the understanding of how and why these foods are the common problems. Connected with food allergy and masking are the ways in which specific alcoholic beverages. and smoking are frequently involved in the whole picture.

Chemical reactions have not been as well documented as food reactions, but to physicians conversant with this new approach they are obvious and important. Many patients are only too aware of their problems with such hydrocarbons as petrol fumes and paint fumes. Until tests have been carried out, patients are usually unaware of the role played by more constantly inhaled chemicals or chemicals in food.

Related to both food and chemical problems is the role of intestinal thrush. This can cause headaches and migraine problems by either predisposing to food or chemical allergies or by a direct weakening effect on the immune system, mediated by the liberation of Candida toxin. There may possibly also be a direct 'allergic-like reaction' to the Candida itself.

Various techniques are discussed which can be used to sort out which factors are operating in individual migraine sufferers. History taking, elimination diets and intradermal provocation testing seem at the moment to be the most useful tools in this respect.

If the patient suffers from many food or chemical allergies, there are likely to be major problems with avoidance. Techniques of neutralization and desensitization to foods and chemicals are described. These procedures immediately enable patients to eat foods to which they are sensitive or inhale chemicals to which they are sensitive without adverse effect. This treatment is either administered by sublingual drops (which protect the patient for five hours) or small subcutaneous injections (self-administered and which protect the patient for two to three days).

There followed proof that neutralization and desensitization are effective and a detailed description of the clinical trials performed in the United States of America and England, which have now conclusively shown that migraine is predominantly a food-allergic disease.

Finally, we explored the factors underlying the occurrence of allergy. As a result of this work, we can point the way to healthier eating habits and lifestyle, which will lessen the chance that allergy will occur in the first place. These findings also help us to understand why allergic manifestations occur at certain times in our life-span and why we may be able to eat commonly-consumed foods for many years before we acquire an adverse reaction to them.

Although I think most migraneurs have the type of underlying causative factors I have discussed, I cannot reconcile the odd case report here and there of the miraculous and permanent cure of migraine by neck manipulation with these factors. I am sure that these reports are genuine and one can only assume that in such patients the problems must stem from a malapposition of the intervertebral joints of the neck. It is curious, however, that the symptoms are so similar to ones produced by allergic manifestations. I can reconcile the frequent help that acupuncture can give migraine sufferers, as acupuncture has been demonstrated to be able to help various allergic diseases. Furthermore, I do have a glimmer of an idea of how this could work.

There are altogether several hundred doctors using the

techniques I have described to help migraine sufferers in the United States of America, Great Britain and Australia. These doctors do not achieve universal success with these methods, but most of their patients lose their migraines and are delighted with their freedom from their 'old enemy'.

Most patients simply have a handful of food allergies and only need these to be identified and usually desensitized. At the other end of the scale are patients beseiged by multiple food and chemical allergies and possibly complicated by a major intestinal thrush problem. These patients, because of the sheer complexity of their disease, pose a major logistic problem with their treatment. Patients with multiple allergies seem to have an unstable immune system. Because of the multiplicity of their reactions, they are very dependent on neutralization/ desensitization therapy but, because of the instability of their immune systems, their neutralizing 'treatment' levels have a nasty habit of changing from time to time. This changeability usually decreases with time. In these complex cases intestinal thrush is usually an underlying factor and treating the thrush seems to decrease the changeability to a large extent.

In other words, most patients who only have a few allergies can be quickly sorted out in a few weeks (and in certain cases in a few days). Patients with very complicated problems may need investigation and treatment extending over several months or even a couple of years before they are well. This new approach to illness, which is best termed clinical ecology, is in my view the most exciting development in medicine since the discovery of antibiotics. Because of its accent on cause and effect as opposed to symptom suppression, it is having problems in gaining acceptance by physicians trained to think only in terms of symptom suppression. There is, however, excellent evidence that it is valid and, as many thousands of patients will testify, it is highly effective and in most of their cases, migraines become a thing of the past. This has become truly a total revolution in the treatment of migraine.

USEFUL ADDRESSES

Action Against Allergy,
43 The Downs,
London SW20 8HG.
Telephone: 01-947 5082
(Mrs A. Nathan-Hill)

This group aims to bring clinical ecology (awareness of food and chemical allergy) to a wider public, and offers many services including: personal information by letter or telephone; postal book service with large selection of books; lending library (for members); films and lectures; information on where to obtain alternative foods, information on the contents of foods and medicines. Please remember to enclose a stamped addressed envelope when writing.

Allergy Support Group, Oxford,
36 Blandford Avenue,
Oxford.
Telephone: (0865) 58931
(Mrs V. Hibbert)

A registered charity and local self-help group. Monthly meetings with medically qualified speakers. Offers information on elimination diets. Their aim is to establish an allergy clinic, preferably NHS. Membership £5 p.a., £1 p.a. for OAPs, students and unwaged.

Cambridge Food Intolerance Society,
1 Gunhild Close,
Cambridge.
Telephone: (0223) 240895
(Mrs B. Stone)

A local self-help group. Meetings with qualified medical speakers approximately six times per year. Membership £3 p.a.

Chemical Victims,
12 Highlands Road,
Worting,
Nr Basingstoke,
Hants.
Telephone: (0256) 65093
(Mrs S. Hedges)

A local self-help group. Monthly meetings and newsletter. Offer information on elimination diets. Membership £5 p.a.

The Fighting Food Allergy Group,
Little Porters,
64a Marshals Drive,
St. Albans,
Herts.
Telephone: (0727) 58705
(Chrys Dowsett)

A local self-help group. Meetings are held once a week, and there is a nominal charge per visit.

Food and Chemical Allergy Association,
27 Ferringham Lane,
Ferring-by-Sea,
West Sussex.
Telephone: (0903) 41178
(Mrs E. Rothera)

Offers personal information by letter or telephone. A pamphlet is available entitled 'Understanding Allergies' (50 pence plus stamped addressed envelope). They do not hold meetings.

Hyperactive Children's Support Group,
59 Meadowside,
Angmering,
Nr Littlehampton,
West Sussex, BN16 4 BW
(Sally Bunday, Secretary/Founder)
No telephone enquiries

This is a national voluntary organization with about 60 local groups, aiming to help the hyperactive child, from the cradle to adolescence. They have various diet sheets available. Please enclose a stamped addressed envelope when writing. The starter diet kit is £2.00 and membership subscription is £3.00

Hythe Food and Chemical Victims' Allergy Club,
44 Fairview Drive,
Hythe,
Southampton.
(Mr J. Spells)
No telephone enquiries

Local self-help group. Monthly meetings and newsletters every three or four months. Membership £2.00 p.a. (£3.00 p.a. for a family). Please write enclosing a stamped addressed envelope.

National Society of Research into Allergy,
PO Box 45,
Hinkley,
Leicester. LE10 1JY
Telephone: (0455) 635212
(Mrs E. Rose)

A national voluntary organization with groups around the country. Elimination diet booklet available. Produces two magazines per year. Meetings held. Offers advice to anyone wishing to set up their own group. Membership £3.00 p.a.

Sanity,
77 Moss Lane,
Pinner,
Middlesex.
(Mrs Margery Hall)
No telephone enquiries

This is a registered charity, which aims to raise funds to further research into the nutritional and biochemical factors in mental illness. Please write enclosing a stamped addressed envelope.

Seaford Food and Chemical Group,
57 Sutton Drive,
Seaford,
Sussex.
Telephone: (0323) 893779
(Mrs R. Jones)

A local self-help group. Monthly meetings and there is a nominal charge per visit. Personal information by telephone (calls taken 9.30-10.30 a.m.)

West Sussex Allergy Group,
28 The Avenue,
Chichester,
West Sussex. PO19 4 PU
Telephone: (0243) 527321
(Mrs A. Shapiro)

A local self-help group. Meetings once a month and there is a nominal charge per visit. Lending library.

Irish Allergy Association,
P.O. Box 1067,
Churchtown,
Dublin. 14

For further information, please write.

FURTHER READING

Chaitow, Leon, *Candida Albicans: Could Yeast be Your Problem?*
(Thorsons, 1985).
Crook, William G., *The Yeast Connection*, obtainable from
author, P.O. Box 3494, Jackson, Tennessee 38301, USA.
Dickey, Lawrence, ed., *Clinical Ecology* (Charles C. Thomas,
1976).
Eagle, Robert, *Eating and Allergy* (Thorsons, 1986).
Hanssen, Maurice, *E for Additives* (Thorsons, 1984).
Mackarness, Richard, *Chemical Victims* (Pan, 1980).
—— *Not All in the Mind* (Pan 1976).
Miller, Joseph B., *Provocative Testing and Injection Therapy*
(Charles C. Thomas, 1972).
Mumby, Keith, *The Food Allergy Plan* (Unwin Paperbacks, 1985).
Nathan-Hill, Amelia, *Against the Unsuspected Enemy* (New
Horizon, 1980).
Randolph, Theron G., and Moss, Ralph W., *Allergies your Hidden
Enemy* (Thorsons, 1984).
Truss, C. Orion, *The Missing Diagnosis*, obtainable from author,
P.O. Box 26508, Birmingham, Alabama 35226, USA.

INDEX

abdominal migraine, 20
  see also pain
acidosis, 51-2
acne, 74, 103
acupuncture and acupressure, 115, 149
adaptation syndrome, the general, 138-9
addiction, 47, 121, 135, 148
  and alcohol, 63-4
  and drugs, 21
  and masking, 25-6
additives, 38, 39-41, 52, 68
agents, bleaching, 52
  emulsifying, 38
air pollution, 41-4, 94-100
alcohol, role of, 62-6, 69
  see also alcoholic beverages
alcoholic beverages, 25, 87, 148
  constituents of, 62-3, 64-6
alcoholism and allergy, 63
allergy
  chemical
    case histories, 54-61
    historical development, 37-43
    Nystatin, 79-80
  definition of, 22-4
  food
    case histories, 54-61
    cyclic and fixed, 28
    diagnosis of, 91-3, 109-14
    as factor in disease, 34-5
    historical development, 22-36
  inhalent 10, 16, 41-3, 94-100, 127
  roots of, 129-42
alternation, 15, 43
animal dander, 94, 105, 110
ankles, swelling of, 20
antibiotics and thrush, 72, 74, 76, 84, 141
antidepressants, 13, 83
anxiety, 125
apples, 38, 39, 65
  see also fruit
arthritis and food allergy, 36
aspirin, 20-1
asthma, 127
Ativan, 83
atmosphere and effect on
  inhaled allergies, 94-5
auto-immune urine therapy, 114-5
avocado pears, 45

avoidance of precipitants, 86-7

background symptoms, 41, 98
Balyeat, Dr R. M., 119
bananas, 37-8, 39
beans, runner, 45, 50
Bentley, Dr D., 128
benzyl alcohol, 88-9
biotin, 81
blood-pressure, abnormal, 20, 54, 126
bowel problems, 72
brassica family and chemicals, 45
bread, 52, 77-8, 134-5
Brostoff, Dr Jonathon, 35, 122, 123, 127, 128
butter, 31, 40

Cafergot, 21, 55
cancer, lung, and smoking, 146-7
Candida albicans see thrush
candidiasis, intestinal
  see thrush
car sickness, 14, 15, 43, 95-6
carbohydrates, 33, 77, 78
Carini, Dr Claudio, 122, 127
carrots, 15, 45, 46, 52
case histories
  allergy, food and chemical 13-17, 54-61, 64
  intradermal testing, 102-4
  thrush, intestinal, 82-5
Catchburian, Dr Adriana, 128
causes of migraine, 9, 85, 148-9
  secondary, 124-5
cereals, 16, 24, 33, 50
  see also under individual names
cheese
  and contraceptive pill, 69
  as precipitant of migraine, 20, 27, 48, 121, 122
  in rotary diet, 30
  and smoking, 66
  and Tyramine, 121
chemical allergy
  historical development of, 37-43
  and Nystatin, 79-80
  see also allergy
chemicals in food, 10
  as root of allergy, 135-7
  solvent, 42
  chlorine, 39-40

chocolate
  and contraceptive pill, 69
  as precipitant of migraine, 20, 27, 48, 121, 122
  and smoking, 66
  and Tyramine, 121
cigarettes, 37, 42, 66, 67, 96, 97, 121
  see also smoking
cigars, 68, 69
citrus fruits, 14, 20, 27, 50, 65, 66, 69, 122
clinical ecology, development of 34-6, 146-7
cluster migraine, 20
Coca, Arthur F., 24, 37
cod, 15, 45, 46
codeine, 20-1
coffee, 25, 39
colourants, 38, 40, 47, 52
confectionary, 40
constipation, 125
Conte, Dr A., 106-7
contraceptive pill
  in case study, 13
  as cause of migraine, 141
  and elimination diet, 47
  and immune system, 69-70, 74-5, 76
  and trials, 66, 121, 122
corn
  as cause of migraine, 134, 148
  and chemical additives, 39
  and diet, 46, 48, 50, 52, 53
  difficulty of avoidance, 65, 86
  and masking, 26, 27, 28
  and testing, 113
cortisone, 75, 76, 138, 139
courgettes, 15, 45, 46
Crook, Dr William, 71, 73
cucumbers, 39
cystitis, 83, 84, 85, 125
cytotoxic testing, 111-12, 113

dander, animal, 94, 105, 110
depression
  case histories, 13, 17, 83, 102
  and elimination diet, 48, 49, 51
  and Nystatin, 79
  as symptom, 20, 125
desensitization therapy, 9, 10, 11, 149, 150
  and case histories, 16, 17, 60, 84
  to foods, 86-93
  and inhaled allergies, 94-100
  intradermal, 56
  and thrush, 81-2
Deseril (methylsergide), 21
DF118, 59
diarrhoea, 82, 125, 126
diet
  cereal-free, 119
  elimination, 44-53
  Feingold, 40
  hypoallergenic, 68, 82, 84
  low-risk, 9-10, 39, 64, 69, 123
  low-tyramine, 121
  monotonous, 134-5
  rotary diversified, 29-32, 35, 56, 119, 135
  and treatment of thrush, 77
  see also elimination diet
    low-risk allergy diet
Dixarit (clonidine hydrochloride), 21, 54, 55
Doerr, Dr, 23
Downing, Dr Damien, 111
drops, sublingual, 16, 17, 90-1
drugs
  addiction to, 21, 47
  antidepressant, 13, 83
  antimigraine, 21
  treatment, 146
  use of, 46, 47, 122

ear infection and food allergy, 36
eczema, 35, 60, 103, 127
eggs, 24-5
  and diagnosis, 86
  and masking, 27, 28
  and rotary diet, 30, 50, 52

Eisenberg, Dr B. C., 120
elimination diet, 44-53
  and case histories, 14, 15, 82
  development of, 23
  and homoeopathy, 116
  and skin-testing, 92
  and tolorance, 28-9
  use of, 10-11, 40-1, 149
empiricalists, 143-6
epidermophyton, 81-2, 137
epilepsy, 126, 127
Epsom salts, 48
ergotamine tartrate, 21, 47, 66, 70, 121, 122
ethanol, synthetic, 43, 95, 99
ethylene gas, 37-8, 39
Eyerman, Dr C. H., 119, 120

families, food, 29, 32, 45, 50, 56, 58, 67
fasting, 27, 44-5
fat, 33
fatigue
  case histories, 13-17
  and chemical allergy, 41, 42
  and elimination diet, 48, 49, 51
  as symptom of migraine, 13, 17, 20
  and thrush, 79, 82, 83
fatty acids, 133-4
Feingold diet, 40
Finn, Dr Ronald, 34, 35, 147
fish, 30, 33, 52
  see also under individual names
flavourings, 29
folic acid, 132
food
  allergy
    case histories, 54-61, 64
    diagnosis of, 91-3, 109-14
    as factor in disease, 34-5
    historical development, 22-36
  families, 29, 32, 45, 50, 56, 58, 67
  low-risk, 45-6
  manufactured, 133
  mixtures, 29, 50
formaldehyde, 37, 97
fruit, 30, 33, 52
  sensitivity to, 38
  see also under individual names
fumes, petrol and diesel, 37, 38, 41, 42-3, 99, 148
  case histories, 15, 82
  treatment, 94-5

gas
  domestic, 41-2, 98-100
  ethylene, 37-8, 39
  phenol, 42
  turpene, 38
gin, 16, 65
glucose, 29, 47
glycerine, 88
Golos, Natalie, 32
Golos-Golbitz, Francis, 32
Gowin, Dr E. L. de, 119, 120
Graham, Dr Pamela, 35
Grant, Dr Ellen
  and oral contraceptives, 74-5
  and symptoms, 125
  trials, 35, 47, 66-7, 69, 70, 118

Hahnemann, Dr Samuel, 115
Hare, Dr Francis, 22
headaches, spectrum of, 20
  types and homoeopathy, 116
Hearn, Dr George, 34
herbs, 31, 65
Herheimer, Dr, 79
Hering, Constantine, 146
Hexheimer reaction, 79, 80, 85
history taking, importance of, 14-15, 40-1, 149
homoeopathy, 115-16
house dust and mite, 84, 94, 110, 127
Hunter, Dr John, 35
Husband, Dr, 34
hydrocarbons, 39, 41-3, 95, 98, 120

hyperactivity, 36, 40, 105, 126
hypertension, 47, 66
hypoallergenic diet, 68, 82, 84

ice-cream, 40
Imipramine, 58
immune system, 148, 150
  and chemicals, 137
  dysfunction, 131-2, 134
  and minerals, 132-3
  and nutrition, 131-2
  and steriods, 69
  and thrush, 73, 75
immunoglobin, 142
inhalant allergies, 10, 16, 41-3, 94-100, 127
injections
  intradermal, 88, 89
  placebo, 89-90, 102-4
  subcutaneous, 16-17, 57, 84, 90-1 102-4
insecticide sprays, 37, 40, 45
Inselman, Dr, 105
Intal, 96
intestinal thrush see thrush
intradermal provocation testing, 15, 88-93, 95,
    99, 101-8, 110, 113, 149
  case studies, 102-4
  see also testing
iron, 132, 133

kerosene, 37
Ketoconazole, 77, 80, 81, 85
kinesiology, applied, 112, 113
King, Dr D., 106
Kingsley, Dr, 34

Lactobacillus acidophilus, 77, 80-1
lactose, 46, 47
lamb, 15, 45, 46
lard, 31
Lee, Dr H. Carlton, 88
Lehman, Dr C., 107
lethargy, 54, 55, 58, 125
Liveing, Dr, 118
Lockey, Dr Stephen, 40
Lomusol, 96
low-risk allergy diet, 9-10, 39, 64, 69, 123
  case histories, 54, 56, 57, 58, 59, 83
low-risk foods, 45-6

Mackarness, Dr Richard, 32-4, 40, 64, 113, 134
malt, 16, 50
Mandell, Dr Marshall, 64, 106-7
margarine, 40
masking, 15, 24-9, 44, 48-9, 63, 68, 148
  and adaptation syndrome, 139
  and addiction, 25-6
  definition of, 25
  importance of, 27
  and trials, 120, 121
meat, 30, 33, 52
  see also under individual names
Megadophilus, 80
membranes, leaky mucous, 73, 141
Migraleave, 54
Migril, 21
milk
  and diagnosis, 86
  and elimination diet, 50, 52, 53
  and masking, 26, 27, 28
  as precipitant of migraine, 121, 134, 148
  and rotary diet, 30
  and testing, 148
Miller, Dr Joseph, 88, 90, 101, 104
minerals, 132-3
Mogadon, 58
monoamine oxide, 121
monosodium glutamate, 52
Monro, Dr Jean, 35, 122, 127
Moss, Dr R. W., 32, 40
moulds, 75, 94, 110, 127, 141
muscle pain (myalgia), 49, 54, 56
  and case histories, 15, 58
myalgia see muscle pain

Nathan-Hill, Amelia, 59-60
nausea, 19, 20, 57, 102, 103
neck manipulation, 149
negative ionizers, 43, 95-6, 97
neutralization therapy, 57, 59, 88-93, 149, 150
  case studies, 102-4
  and intradermal testing, 101-8
  and thrush, 73
Nizoral (Ketoconazole), 77, 80, 81, 85
nutrition, 10, 130-2, 141
nuts, 31
Nystatin, 72, 77, 78-80, 81, 82-3, 84, 85

oats, 16, 31, 50, 65
obesity see weight problems
oil, 15, 31, 86
  domestic, 41, 98-100
  and gas deposits, 38
  see also gas
oleic acid, 81
oral contraceptives see
  contraceptive pill
oranges, 27, 30
O'Shea, Dr James, 105

pain
  abdominal, 59, 125, 126
  chest, 82, 83
  muscle, 15, 49, 54, 56, 58
painkillers, 20-1
paint, 37, 42, 97, 99, 148
palpitations, 20, 83
pantothenic acid, 132
paracetamol, 20-1
paraffin wax, 39
parsnips, 15, 45
pathology, preoccupation
  with, 146
pears, 15, 45, 46
pepper, green, 39
perfumes, 37, 41, 97, 99
period and headaches, 13, 57, 125
pesticides, 37, 40, 45
Peters, Dr Dale, 143
pethidine, 103
petrochemicals, 37, 94
  see also fumes
petrol fumes see fumes
phenol (soft plastic), 42, 97, 98
phenolic resin, 52
pill see contraceptive pill
Pirquet, Clement von, 22-3
pituitary gland, 139
placebo, 89-90, 105, 106, 107, 123, 127
plaice, 45, 46
plastics, soft, 42, 97, 98
pollens, 94, 110
pollution, 41-3, 94-100
Porter, Dr S. F., 105
potassium bicarbonate, 51
potatoes, 39, 50, 52
Pottenger Cat Studies, 129-31
preservatives, 38, 52
prick testing, 88, 109-10
primitive foods, 33
protein, 30, 33
psychological symptoms, 106
pyridoxine, 132

Radcliffe, Dr, 34
radionics, 112-13
Randolph, Dr Theron G., 28, 32, 33, 37, 119, 120
  and chemical sensitivity, 38, 40, 95
Rapp, Dr Doris, 126
RAST test (radio allergo sorbent test) 110-11,
    123-3, 128
rationalists, 143-6
Rea, Dr William J., 104, 136-7
rectal irritation, 84
resistance and adaptation as root of allergy,
    138-42
rhinitis, 24-5, 49, 82, 83, 126-7

Rinkel, Dr Herbert, 24-6, 28, 37, 49, 119
  see also Rinkel's hyperacute response
Rinkel's hyperacute response, 25, 27, 39, 49, 146
  see also Rinkel, Dr Herbert
rotary diversified diet, 29-32, 35, 56, 119, 135
Rowe, Albert, 23, 24, 37, 119, 120
royal free disease, 140
rye, 16, 31, 50, 65

saccharine, 52
Saiffer, Dr Phyllis, 87-8
salmon, 15
salt, 15, 29, 46
Schiff, Dr Boris, 105
scotch, 16, 65
seeds, 31
selenium, 132, 133
Selye, Hans, 138
Shapiro, Dr R. S., 120
Sheldon, Dr J. M., 37, 119, 120
shellfish, 30
side-effects, 21, 116
skin testing, 16, 91-3, 132
  see also testing
smoking, role of, 47, 66-9, 146-7,
  see also cigarettes
sodium bicarbonate, 48, 51, 77
sodium cromoglycate (Nalcrom), 58, 59, 96, 97,
  98, 127-8
soft drinks, 40
solanaceae food family, 67
solpadeine, 20-1
solvent chemicals, 42
Soothill, Professor, 9, 35, 118, 126
soya, 29, 46, 50, 52, 53
  as food constituent, 134-5
spices, 31
spirits, 14
  see also alcohol
sponge rubber, 42
starch, 29
steroids, 69, 74-5
stress, 13, 42, 138, 140
sublingual provocation testing, 113-14
  trials, 106-8
  see also testing
sugar
  and elimination diet, 46, 47, 50, 52-3
  and masking, 25, 27, 28
  as precipitant of migraine, 33, 65, 86, 134, 141,
    148
  and smoking, 67-8
  and thrush, 76, 77
sulphur dioxide, 39
Superdophilus, 80-1
swedes, 15, 45
sweeteners, 31
symptoms of migraine, 19-20
  associated 125-8
  see also case histories

tar, 97
TCE, 81-2
tea, 25, 31
testing
  cytotoxic, 111-12, 113
  and diagnosis, 91-3
  intradermal provocation, 15, 88-93, 95, 99,
    101-8, 110, 113, 149
  kinesiology, 112, 113
  prick, 88, 109-10
  RAST, 110-11, 122-3, 128
  sublingual provocation, 113,14, 106-8
tetracycline, 74
Thompson, Jenny (case history), 13-17
thrombophlebitis, 36
thrush, 29, 47, 72-85
  Candida toxin, 73, 74, 79, 141, 148
  case histories, 60, 82-3
  causes of, 73
  and chemical problems, 85
  and contraceptive pill, 69-70
  diagnosis of, 74

diet, importance of, 77
and food allergy, 32, 73, 74, 114
and mould, 75, 78, 81
mycelial fungal form, 72, 81
predisposing factors to, 75-6, 77, 78
as root of allergy, 129, 137-8, 141, 148, 150
symptoms of, 76-7
and yeast, 75-6, 77, 78
yeast-like form, 72, 81
tinnitus, 102
tobacco, 25, 68, 69
  see also smoking
tolerance, food, 28-9, 135
tolune in paint, 97
treatment, 43, 149
  current drug, 20-1
  of food allergies, 114-17
trials
  double-blind, 34, 35, 102, 104
  migraine, 118-28
  neutralization therapy, 101-5
  sublingual provocation, 106-8
trichophyton, 81-2, 137
trout, 15, 45, 46
Truss, Dr Orion, 71, 72, 73, 83
turnips, 15, 45
tyramine, 121

ulcers, mouth, 59, 60, 127
Unger, Dr A. H., 119, 120
Unger, Dr L., 119, 120
ureaformaldehyde foam, 97
urine, 114-5

vaginitis, 72, 84, 85, 127
Valium, 58, 64
varnish, 41, 97
Vaughan, Dr W. T., 118
vegetables, 30, 33, 37, 38, 52
  see also under individual names
visual disturbance, 19-20, 55, 57
vitamins, 132, 133
vodka, 64-5
vomiting, 19, 20, 57, 59, 103

water
  spring, 15, 39, 40, 44, 46, 51
  tap, 39, 51
weight problems
  in case histories, 13, 14, 16, 54, 58, 83, 84
  and fasting, 44
  and primitive foods, 33
  as symptom of migraine, 20, 125
Weindorf, Dr, 105
wheals
  bound, 90
  duitero, 90
  negative, 89, 95, 106, 110
  positive, 89, 91, 95, 99, 106
  and testing, 114
wheat
  avoidance of, 86, 65
  and elimination diet, 46, 50, 52, 53
  as precipitant of migraine, 134, 148
  and testing, 113
whole foods, 29
Williams, Roger J., 133
wine, 14, 20, 27, 62, 65-6, 121
  see also alcohol
withdrawal reaction, 15, 16, 26, 28, 48-9
  case histories, 54, 55, 57, 58, 60, 83
  and coffee, 115-16

yeast
  avoidance of, 86
  and elimination diet, 46, 50, 52, 53
  and masking, 26, 29
  as precipitant of migraine, 64, 65, 134, 141
  and rotary diet, 31
  and thrush, 75-6, 77, 78

Zeller, Michael, 28, 37
Zilka, Dr K., 122
zinc, 132, 133